Editor: David Barlex

*Teacher's Guide*
Authors: David Barlex with Jo Compton

*Capability Task File*
Authors: Jill Bancroft, Eileen Barlex, Maria Cavadino, Lucy Golding,
Marion Rutland, Jane Sharp, Sue Smeaton
Illustrations: Russell Birkett

Addison Wesley Longman Limited
Edinburgh Gate, Harlow, Essex, CM20 2JE
© The Nuffield Foundation 1996

First published in 1996
ISBN 0 582 29071 6

Design by Linda Males
Printed by Pindar plc
Set in Minion 12/15pt

The Publishers' policy is to use paper manufactured from sustainable forests.

# Contents

## Part 2 Capability Tasks for 14–16 year-olds

### Food products for special diets

### Food products for the very young

### Food products for the elderly

### Food products for those at risk

### Food products from primary foods

### Food products from the bakery

### Food products from a confectioner

# Part 1

## Teaching D&T to 14–16 year-olds

The Nuffield approach to design and technology has proved extremely successful. At the time of writing, it is being used by over one third of the secondary schools in England and Wales. It is quite clear that the Nuffield Project's slogan 'Teaching students to design what they are going to make and then make what they have designed' is no idle boast. These materials have been designed to build on this proven approach, but it is important to note that a school can use the materials 'from scratch' with students who have not met the approach previously. By using the approach and the associated materials, schools will be able to meet the requirements of the 1995 Statutory Orders for design and technology and prepare students for a variety of different Examination Board syllabuses. Quite deliberately, the Nuffield approach is not allied to any one Examination Board but the Nuffield Project has worked closely with a number of different Examination Boards and this guide describes how the materials can be used to meet different Examination Board requirements. The Teacher's Guide deals with the area of design and technology most commonly called Food Technology. The publications for this area are shown below.

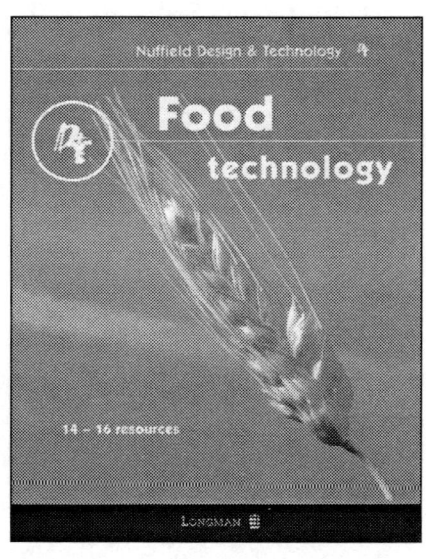

### Food Technology Student's Book

A complete textbook to support the pupils in producing course work, learning the substance of design and technology, and tackling written examinations. You will need class sets with, ideally, each pupil having access to their own copy.

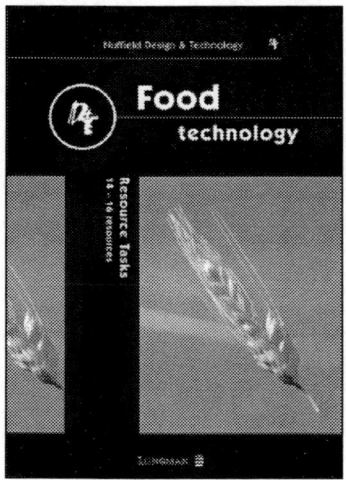

### Food Technology Resource Tasks File

This is a once only purchase containing over 30 focused practical tasks as copymasters. Through these tasks you can teach the content required for GCSE success.

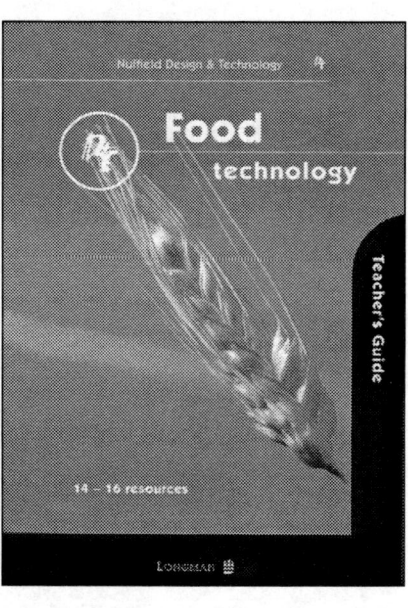

### Food Technology Teacher's Guide

This is a once only purchase. Part 1 explains how to use the published materials and approach to construct a scheme of work suitable for your school and Examination Board. Part 2 contains 12 different Capability Tasks.

If you teach design and technology the Nuffield way, then you will use three different teaching methods.

- **Resource Tasks.** These are short, practical activities. They have been designed to make students think and help them learn the knowledge and skills they need to design and make things really well.

- **Case Studies.** These are true stories about design and technology in the world outside school. By reading them students find out more than they possibly could through designing and making alone. Through Case Studies they will learn about the way firms and businesses design and manufacture goods and how those goods are marketed and sold. They will also learn about the impact that products make on the people who use them and the places where they are made.

- **Capability Tasks.** These involve designing and making a product that works. Students use what they have learned in Resource Tasks and Case Studies when they tackle a Capability Task. Capability Tasks take a lot longer than either Resource Tasks or Case Studies. You will need to organize your lessons so that students do the Resource Tasks and Case Studies they need for a Capability Task as part of that Capability Task. That way you can make sure that your students can be successful in their designing and making.

The way these methods work together is shown here in this extract from the Student's Book.

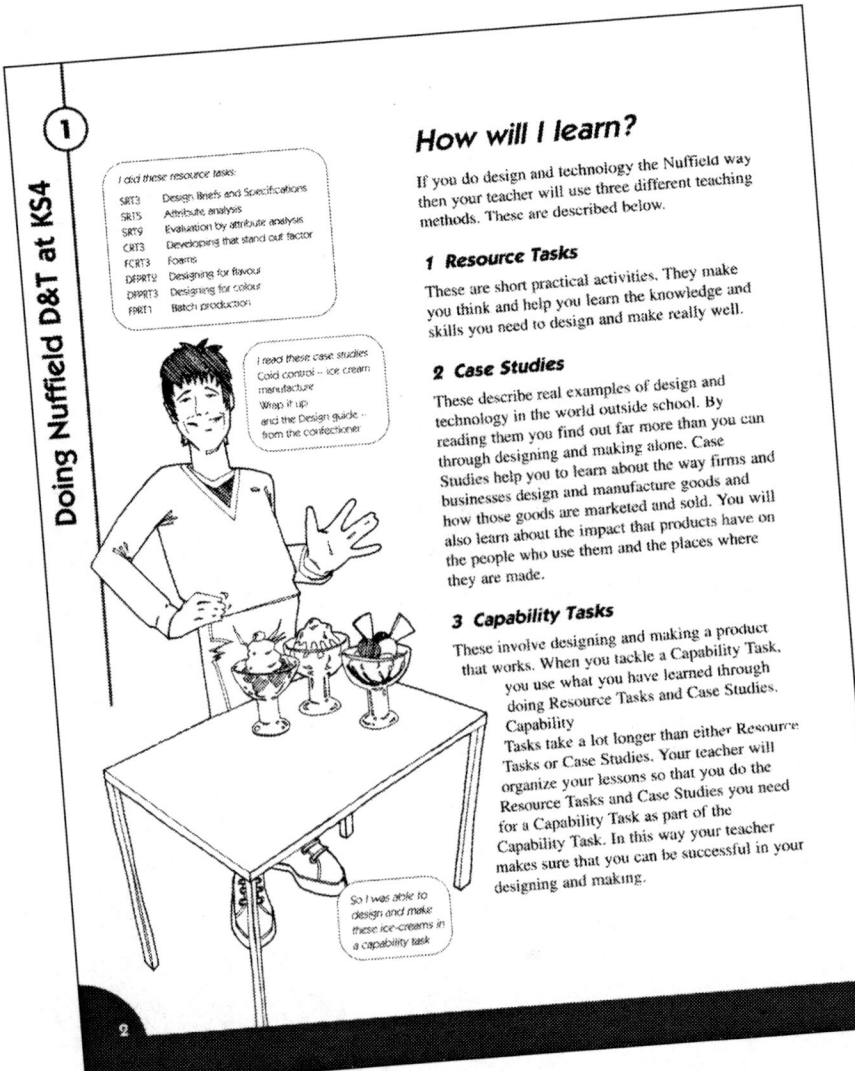

## A new design for 14–16 year-olds

Each Resource Task is presented to the student as an instruction sheet laid out like this.

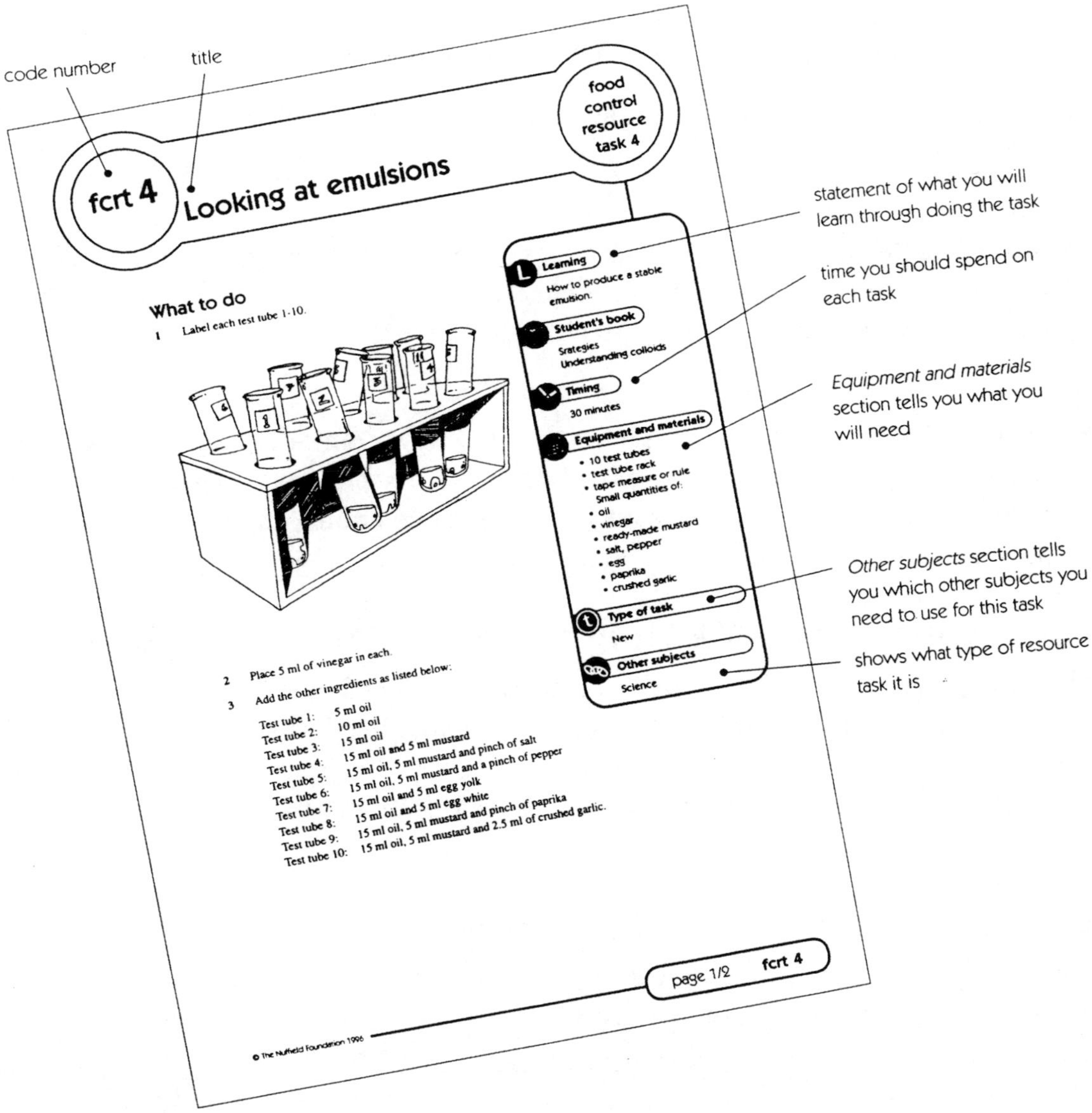

code number · · · title

**fcrt 4** Looking at emulsions

food control resource task 4

**What to do**

1 Label each test tube 1-10.

**L Learning**
How to produce a stable emulsion.

statement of what you will learn through doing the task

**Student's book**
Strategies
Understanding colloids

**Timing**
30 minutes

time you should spend on each task

**Equipment and materials**
• 10 test tubes
• test tube rack
• tape measure or rule
Small quantities of:
• oil
• vinegar
• ready-made mustard
• salt, pepper
• egg
• paprika
• crushed garlic

Equipment and materials section tells you what you will need

**Type of task**
New

**Other subjects**
Science

Other subjects section tells you which other subjects you need to use for this task

shows what type of resource task it is

2 Place 5 ml of vinegar in each.

3 Add the other ingredients as listed below:

Test tube 1: 5 ml oil
Test tube 2: 10 ml oil
Test tube 3: 15 ml oil
Test tube 4: 15 ml oil and 5 ml mustard
Test tube 5: 15 ml oil, 5 ml mustard and a pinch of salt
Test tube 6: 15 ml oil, 5 ml mustard and a pinch of pepper
Test tube 7: 15 ml oil and 5 ml egg yolk
Test tube 8: 15 ml oil and 5 ml egg white
Test tube 9: 15 ml oil, 5 ml mustard and pinch of paprika
Test tube 10: 15 ml oil, 5 ml mustard and 2.5 ml of crushed garlic.

page 1/2 fcrt 4

The design is different from that used earlier. While still incorporating its key features, it has two additional features appropriate for 14–16 year olds. These are an indication of the type of task (see page 4) and the links with other subjects.

You may organize the lesson so that everyone is doing the same Resource Task, set different students different tasks or allow them to choose from a range of Resource Tasks. Sometimes the tasks require students to work on their own and sometimes as part of a team.

Chapters 5 to 12 of the *Food Technology Student's Book* contain cross-references to Resource Tasks (see below) showing that the information on this page will be useful in tackling the Resource Task indicated.

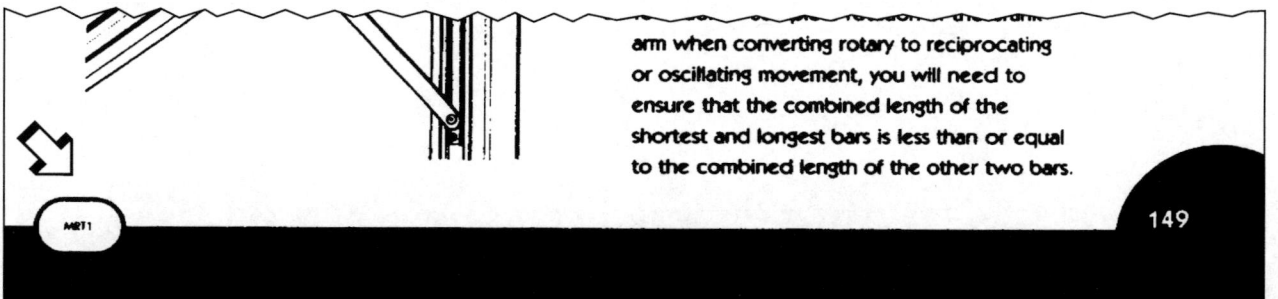

arm when converting rotary to reciprocating or oscillating movement, you will need to ensure that the combined length of the shortest and longest bars is less than or equal to the combined length of the other two bars.

MRT1

## ③ Types of Resource Task

There are three basic types of Resource Tasks.

- **Recapitulation Resource Tasks.** These are tasks that go over things that students probably did earlier. They are very useful for reminding students of things they may have forgotten about or for catching up on things they have missed.

- **Extension Resource Tasks.** These are tasks that take an idea that students were probably taught earlier and develop it further. They are useful for both revising ideas explored earlier and helping students use them in a more advanced way.

- **New ideas Resource Tasks.** These are tasks that deal with knowledge and understanding that are new to 14–16 year-olds. It is unlikely that students will have done this sort of work earlier. They are important for helping the students make progress.

You can use this classification in a number of useful ways. You can organize the sequence of Resource Tasks in a way that shows students the progress they can make by working through them. Students who are facing difficulties can spend longer on recapitulation tasks. Particularly able students can miss out recapitulation tasks altogether.

## Style and range of learning through Resource Tasks

The style of learning is **active**. It always involves a response from the student.

Students might have to explain, record, design, construct, investigate or test. The learning intentions for any one Resource Task are likely to be quite narrow, but, where possible, tasks have been written that meet several learning intentions. In this way Resource Tasks can be used very efficiently.

## The substance of the Resource Tasks

The Resource Tasks are divided into nine sets as shown in Table 1. Five of these sets are developments from earlier Resource Tasks and there are four categories new for 14–16 year-olds – 'Food chemistry', 'Designing food products', 'Food production' and 'Food sales'. Through the Food chemistry tasks, students will be able to investigate setting, foams and emulsions and also carry out simple food tests. Through the Designing food products tasks, students will gain experience in designing to achieve particular requirements in flavour, colour, texture, finish, shelf-life, cost and nutrition. The Food production tasks teach students about batch production and the importance of controlling conditions in products that are produced using biochemical reactions. The Food sales tasks deal with the areas of food hygiene and food product labelling.

You can find a detailed summary of all the Food Technology Resource Tasks on pages 36–38.

## Table 1 – Food technology Resource Tasks

| Strategies | Communicating | Designing food products |
|---|---|---|
| SRT 1 Identifying needs and likes | CRT 1 Presenting information about food products | DFPRT 1 Designing for nutrition |
| SRT 2 Questionnaires | CRT 2 Exploring packaging | DFPRT 2 Designing for flavour and aroma |
| SRT 3 Design briefs and specifications | CRT 3 Developing that 'stand out' factor | DFPRT 3 Designing for colour |
| SRT 4 Brainstorming | CRT 4 Communicating production methods | DFPRT 4 Designing for texture |
| SRT 5 Attribute analysis | | DFPRT 5 Designing for finish |
| SRT 6 Evaluating using ranking, preference and difference tests | | DFPRT 6 Designing for shelf-life |
| SRT 7 Winners and losers and appropriateness | | DFPRT 7 Designing for cost |
| SRT 8 User trip and performance specification | | |
| SRT 9 Evaluation by attribute profile | | |

| Food chemistry | Nutrition | Food production |
|---|---|---|
| FCRT 1 Food tests | NRT 1 What's in food | FPRT 1 Batch production and systems thinking |
| FCRT 2 Making things set | NRT 2 Changing the nutritional value of food products | FPRT 2 Biotechnology in the food industry |
| FCRT 3 Looking at foams | | |
| FCRT 4 Looking at emulsions | | |

| Food sales | Products and applications | Health and safety |
|---|---|---|
| FSRT 1 Breaking the chain | PART 1 Comparing a collection of food products | HSRT 1 Ensuring safety in an unfamiliar situation |
| FSRT 2 Labelling: who needs it? | | |

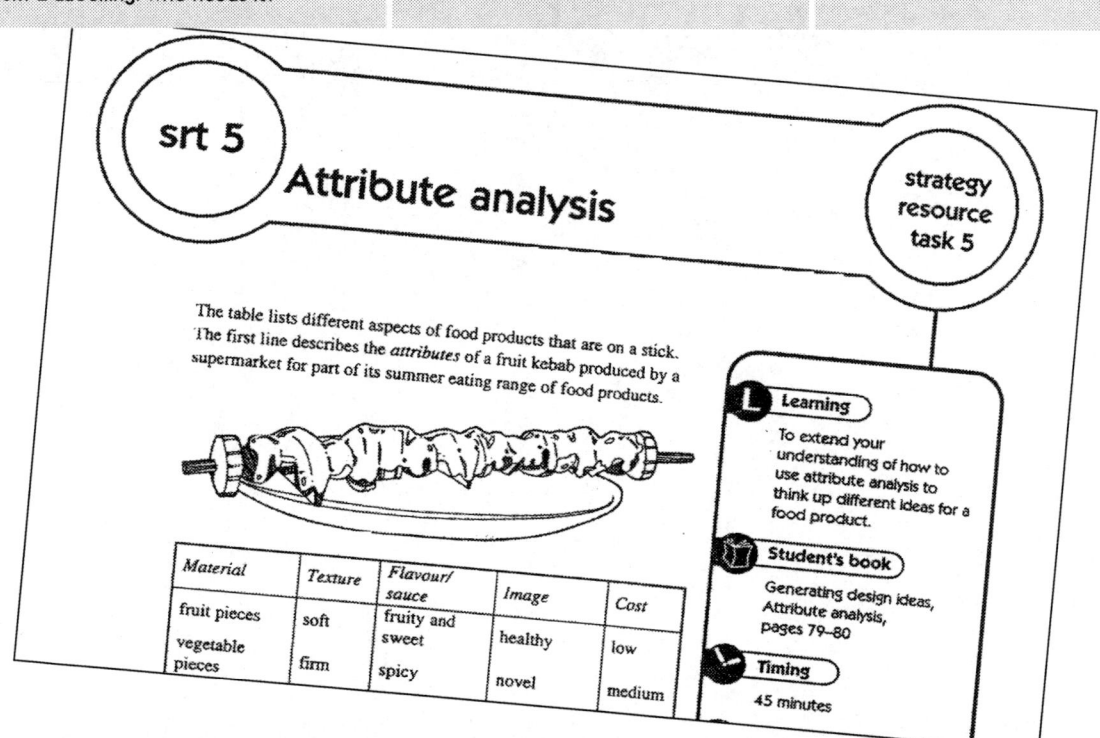

srt 5

# Attribute analysis

strategy resource task 5

The table lists different aspects of food products that are on a stick. The first line describes the *attributes* of a fruit kebab produced by a supermarket for part of its summer eating range of food products.

**Learning**

To extend your understanding of how to use attribute analysis to think up different ideas for a food product.

**Student's book**

Generating design ideas, Attribute analysis, pages 79–80

**Timing**

45 minutes

| Material | Texture | Flavour/sauce | Image | Cost |
|---|---|---|---|---|
| fruit pieces | soft | fruity and sweet | healthy | low |
| vegetable pieces | firm | spicy | novel | medium |

# ③ Organizing the classroom

Following these guidelines will help ensure that Resource Task work is effective.

- Each student should have a copy of the instruction sheets.

- Each student should have a separate copy of any tables or worksheets required to be filled in during the task. Make sure that some spares are available for mistakes.

- Allow sufficient time and, if necessary, deviate from the recommended time.

- Ensure that the required materials, tools and equipment are readily available.

- Use a circus approach within your classroom to avoid equipment shortfalls.

- If necessary, go through the task with the class beforehand so that all students have clear targets for doing and recording.

- If necessary, demonstrate skills that will be needed for the task.

- If you require the students to tackle a sequence of Resource Tasks over successive lessons, share this with the class.

- Once the students are tackling the task, support them by asking questions, giving assistance, looking at what they write and draw, helping with practical difficulties and providing encouragement.

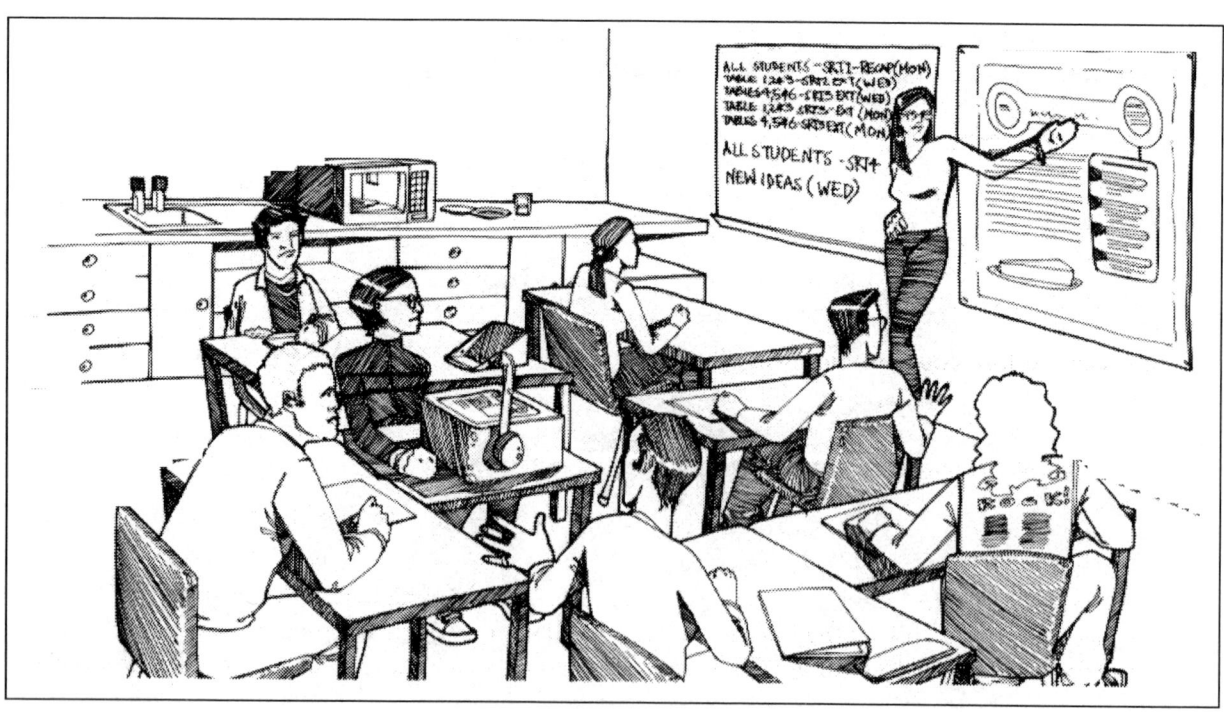

*A teacher sets up a sequence of Resource Tasks over successive lessons and goes through the first task.*

The *Student's Book* provides support for all aspects of GCSE courses. All *Student's Books* have the same overall structure, ensuring continuity of treatment whatever the focus area. The purpose and key features of each section of the *Food Technology Student's Book* are described below.

## Chapter 1 Doing Nuffield D&T for 14–16 year-olds

This chapter is divided into three parts.

### Part 1 Learning D&T for 14–16 year-olds

This gives a clear description of the sorts of products that students will design and make during their course, plus an explanation of the Nuffield approach. The use of Resource Tasks, Capability Tasks and Case Studies is described and there is guidance on reviewing progress during a Capability Task, evaluating the final product and assessing overall progress.

### Part 2 Using other subjects in D&T

This identifies ways students can use art, science, mathematics and information technology to enhance designing and making.

### Part 3 How you will be assessed at GCSE

This gives guidance on how to develop and carry out a Capability Task for GCSE course work and how to research and write a Case Study for GCSE course work. It also describes four types of questions used for GCSE written, terminal examinations.

You can use this part of the *Student's Book* as the basis for whole-class teaching about the way students will learn and as a basis for helping individual students with particular difficulties. For example, you might ask a student to read the section on using science and identify some science that he or she has been taught earlier if they are tackling a Capability Task in which science is likely to be useful. This could become the basis for the student talking to both their science and D&T teachers about ways in which the science could be applied.

## Chapter 2 Exam questions

A range of exam questions, approved by SCAA, and typical of those likely to be set for GCSE written, terminal examinations is presented with comments.

## Chapter 3 Case Studies

There are two sorts of Case Studies. First, a set that is common to all the *Student's Books*, whatever the focus area. These deal with the technologies that really affect the way people live. Often they are associated with a particular time in history. Reading these will help students understand the way that technology affects our lives. Second, there are those that deal with products that are similar to those that the students will be designing and making. They will describe the following about these products:

- how the designs were developed, manufactured, marketed and sold;

- how the products work;

- how the products affect people, those who make it, those who use it and others.

A particular study may deal with just one of these or it may describe all of them. By reading these studies, students will gain an insight into professional practice that will inform their own designing and making.

There are two devices to help students read the studies. First, 'Pause for thought' features that ask intriguing questions but do not require the reader to write anything down. They are there to provide motivation to read more. Second, there are 'questions' to answer. You can use these as staging posts for reading a Case Study as a class activity. For example, you could instruct the class as follows: 'I want you to spend 15 minutes reading this Case Study and discussing the questions with your partner. Then I want you to answer the questions in writing. This should take you a further ten minutes'. The Case Studies also contain 'Research activity'. You can set these for homework as they involve finding out information that is not in the Case Study. The titles of the Case Studies are shown in Table 2.

You can find details of the links between the Case Studies and Capability Tasks in the table on pages 40–44.

## Table 2 – Food technology Case Studies

| General case studies | Focus case studies |
| --- | --- |
| Designing our surroundings | Wrap it up |
| Information – the power to change lives | Soup, beautiful soup |
| DIY medical testing | A corny story |
| Manufacturing aircraft | Copper and you |
| Public transport in London | Breadmaking in Peru |
| Technological endeavours | Brand names for sweeties |
| | Bread production |
| | Making minced meat |
| | Energy to make things work |
| | Embedded energy |
| | Cool control |

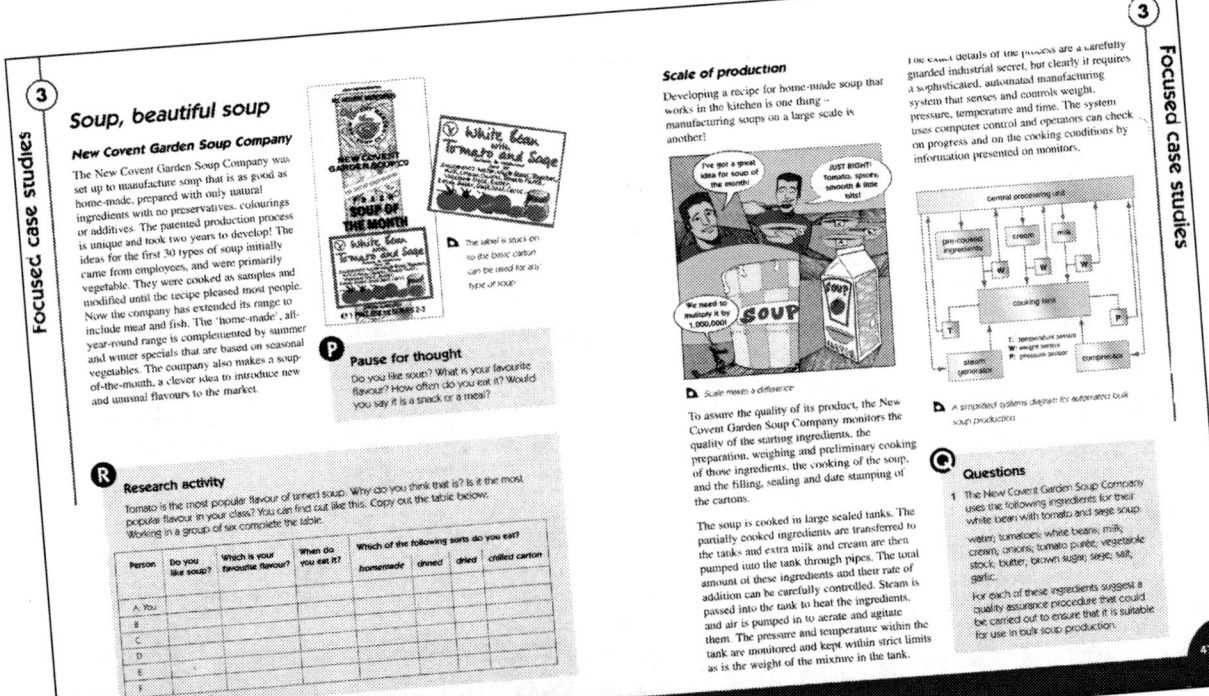

# Chapter 4 Strategies

This chapter revisits and develops strategies from earlier and introduces some new ones for 14–16 year-olds. The strategies are shown in Table 3. The aim of this chapter is to provide the student with a repertoire of strategies and sufficient understanding to be able to choose and use them appropriately.

## Table 3 – Strategies for 14–16 year-olds

| Strategies | Strategies |
|---|---|
| Identifying needs and likes | Applying science |
|     thinking about what people might need |     understanding colloids |
|     observing people |     understanding the nutrition–respiration relationship |
|     asking questions | Systems thinking |
|     using books and magazines |     user and operator interfaces |
|     image boards |     a closer look at feedback and control |
|     using questionnaires | Planning |
| Design briefs |     flow charts and Gantt charts |
| Specifying the product | Evaluating |
| Generating design ideas |     user trip |
|     brainstorming |     winners and losers |
|     observational drawing |     ranking tests |
|     attribute analysis |     difference tests |
| Defining and refining food product ideas |     preference tests |
| Using computers |     evaluation by attribute profile |
| |     performance testing |
| |     is it appropriate? |

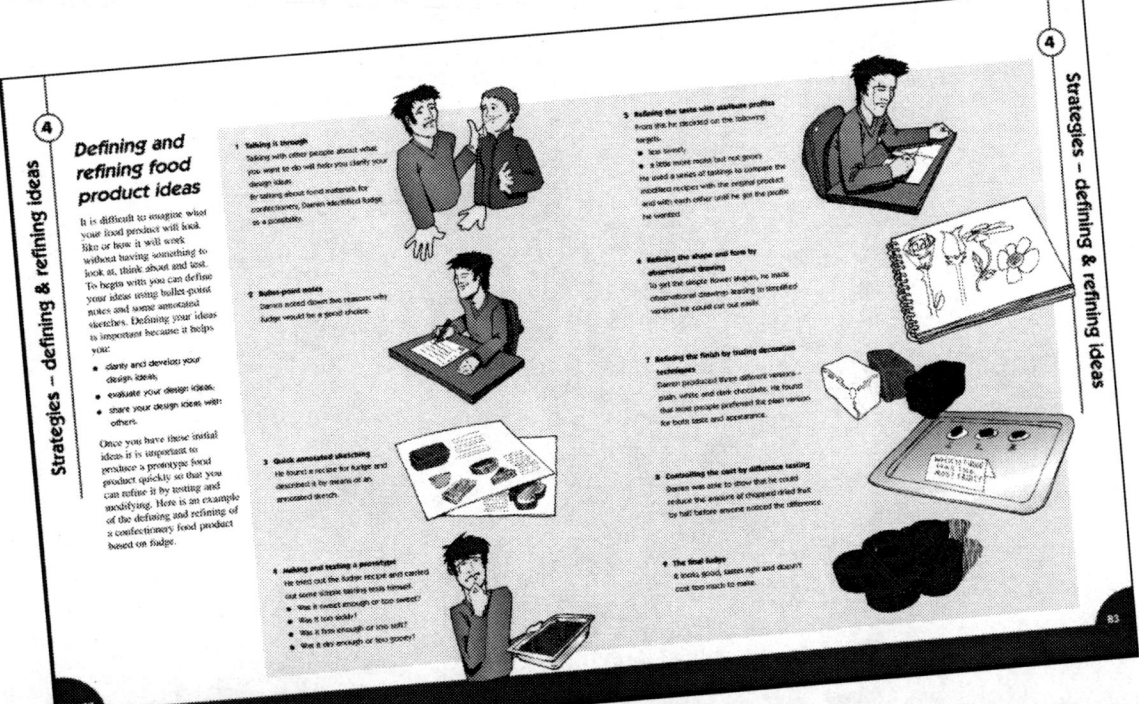

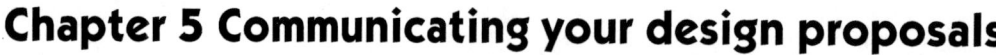
# Chapter 5 Communicating your design proposals

This chapter builds on the earlier approaches in detailing the techniques used by designers to communicate with both the client and the manufacturer. The aim of this chapter is to enable the student to choose and use techniques that are appropriate for the information to be conveyed. Table 4 summarizes the techniques and purposes dealt with in this chapter.

## Table 4 – Communication techniques for 14–16 year-olds

| What you want to communicate | Techniques to use |
| --- | --- |
| what the product looks like | slides and photographs |
| what the product tastes like | taste presentation |
| what others think of the taste | results of sensory analysis testing |
| attractive appearance when on sale | suitable packaging:<br><br>• producing mock-ups<br><br>• evaluating against competitors |
| legally required information | clear listing according to EU regulations |
| how to make a prototype | recipe |
| how to produce with quality assurance | production schedule |
| industrial production with quality assurance | industrial production schedule |
| how to use the product | on pack information:<br><br>• cooking instructions<br><br>• storage instructions<br><br>• associated recipes |

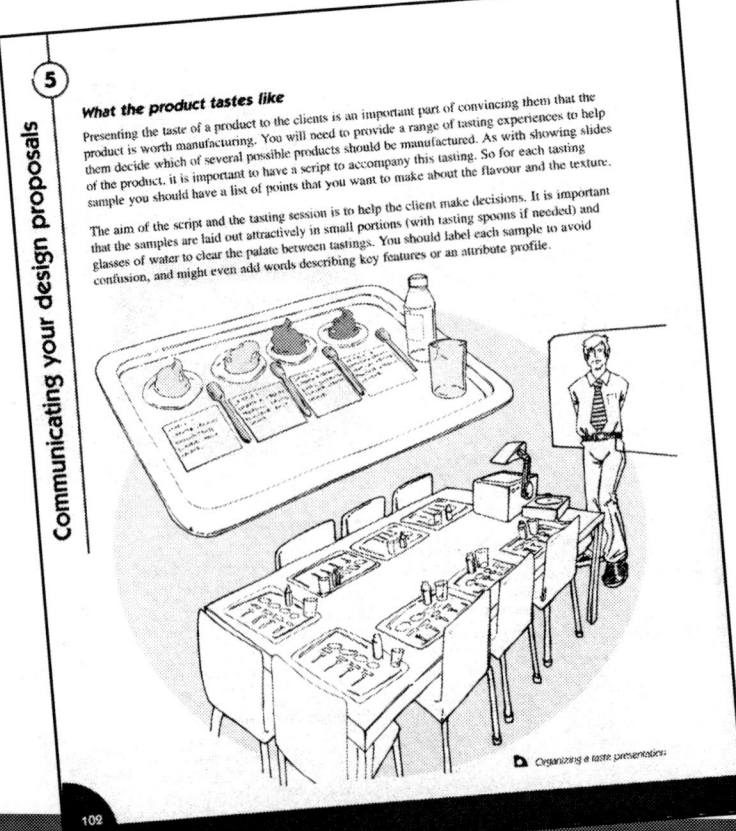

**What the product tastes like**

Presenting the taste of a product to the clients is an important part of convincing them that the product is worth manufacturing. You will need to provide a range of tasting experiences to help them decide which of several possible products should be manufactured. As with showing slides of the product, it is important to have a script to accompany this tasting. So for each tasting sample you should have a list of points that you want to make about the flavour and the texture.

The aim of the script and the tasting session is to help the client make decisions. It is important that the samples are laid out attractively in small portions (with tasting spoons if needed) and glasses of water to clear the palate between tastings. You should label each sample to avoid confusion, and might even add words describing key features or an attribute profile.

Organizing a taste presentation.

# Chapter 6 Design guides

The Nuffield Project has developed the idea of a line of interest as a means of limiting the sorts of product that students in a class might design and make. This makes the teaching of a capability task much more manageable. A line of interest describes a particular type of product and the Nuffield Project has suggested the following seven lines of interest as being suitable for food technology:

- food products for special diets
- food products for the very young
- food products for the elderly
- food products for those at risk
- food products from primary foods
- food products from the bakery
- food products from a confectioner.

Chapter 6 contains a design guide for each of these lines of interest and each guide deals with the issues that should be considered when designing within this line of interest. They set an agenda for the students rather than providing the answers. They are all presented in a similar way using the same set of headings.

- 'What are the important background facts?'
- 'What types of product do they sell already?' or 'What is already on the market?'
- 'What types of products might they develop?'
- 'What are the nutritional needs?' or 'What are the nutritional issues?'; and for particular groups of people, 'What is their situation?'

In addition, there is a resources checklist that summarizes knowledge and understanding of the problem, for the solution and useful strategies.

The design guides provide a straightforward way for students to become familiar with areas of food technology. They can act as a stimulus for students who are having difficulty in deciding on their main course work. They can provide a reminder during a capability task, ensuring that important issues are not overlooked. You can use the design guides in a number of ways.

- In one-to-one conversations with individual students, as in 'I'm not sure that you've thought about all the important things here; let's look at the design guide to see if you've missed anything'.

- In conversations with small groups, as in 'I want you to use the design guide to find four questions to ask each other about your design ideas. I'll be back in ten minutes to see how you're getting on.'

- In a question and answer session with the whole class, as in 'It says here that there is an increase in vegetarian consumers. Hands up who thinks that's true. Most of you? OK, Jane, I want you to tell the class why you believe this is true and, then, Paul, I want you to give me two examples of vegetarian products and where they can be bought.'

- As reading homework in preparation for a Capability Task that you can build on with a question and answer session the following lesson.

# Chapter 7 Food chemistry

This chapter builds on the introductory earlier work, describing the composition and structure of the compounds in the major food groups. It then discusses the food chemistry underlying important cooking and food preparation processes. Finally, it describes a range of simple tests for food materials that students can carry out in school science laboratories. The contents are summarized in Table 5.

The aim of this chapter is to enable students to adopt a rational approach to recipe modification and new product development. By using the information here, students should be able to decide on a course of action and justify it.

## Table 5 – Food chemistry for 14–16 year-olds

| Why is food chemistry important? | Food chemistry in action |
|---|---|
| **What's in food?** | How can I get food to go brown? |
| Composition of carbohydrates | caramelization |
| glucose | Maillard reaction |
| starch | How can I make my mixture set? |
| cellulose | protein sets |
| Composition of fats | effect of overheating on protein set |
| glycerol | starch sets |
| fatty acids | How can I make a mixture light and fluffy in texture? |
| saturated fatty acids | Get liquids to stay mixed |
| polyunsaturated fatty acids | **Food tests** |
| Composition of protein | Testing for sugars |
| essential and non-essential amino acids | Testing for starch |
| sequence of amino acids in chain | Testing for fats |
| | Testing for vitamin C |
| | Testing for protein |

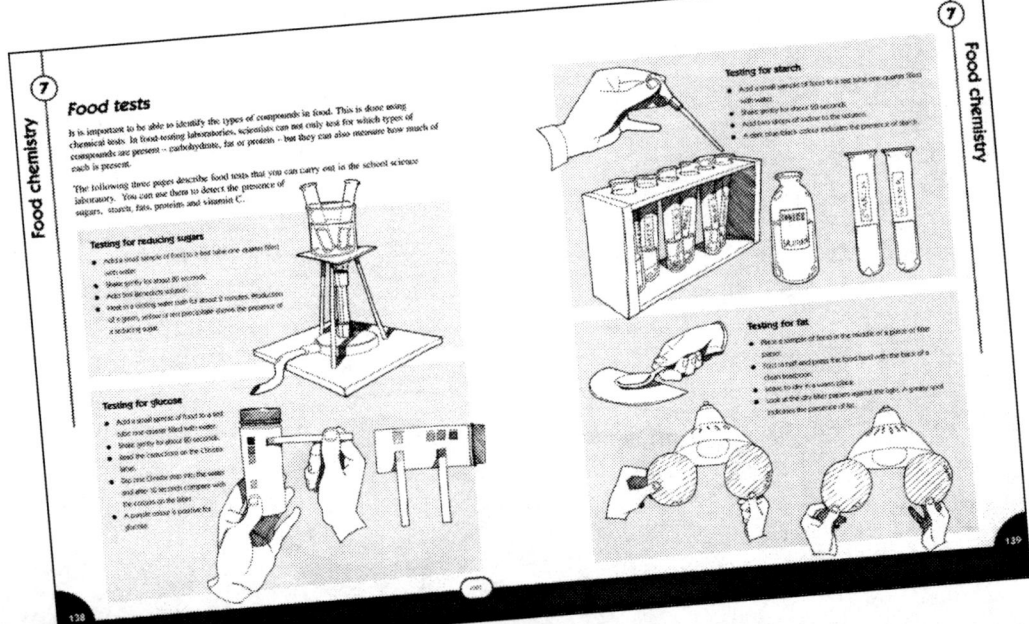

# Chapter 8 Nutrition

This chapter builds on earlier introductory work. It begins by describing digestion in terms of enzyme action at different points in the alimentary canal. It describes the role of dietary fibre and discusses dietary needs. It revisits the functions of the nutrients in food and summarizes the ways in which nutritional information is given (Dietary Reference Values, Reference Nutrient Intake and Estimated Average Requirements). It discusses the relationship between energy intake and obesity. It describes three conditions affected by diet – coronary heart disease, dental caries and diabetes – and discusses the eating disorders bulimia and anorexia nervosa.

# Chapter 9 Food product design

This chapter is divided into seven sections, each of which deals with an important aspect of food product design.

## Designing for nutrition

This section begins by giving examples of cultural variations in nutrition and then presents basic nutritional information as a series of chooser charts in which the nutritional content of different food materials is described by means of a blob score.

These charts have been developed to provide students with a rapid approach to considering nutritional values and to help with decision making about the nutritional content of a food product on a broad sweep basis. For detailed work, students must, of course, consult food value tables with numerical data.

A selection of pie charts is presented to show that all the nutritional information for a food material may be presented visually.

Finally, the effect of cooking methods on nutritional values is discussed.

## Designing for flavour and odour

This section uses the idea of spectrum of intensity – from 'strong', 'powerful' or 'pungent' to 'medium', 'weak' or 'mild', ending with 'subtle', 'faint' or 'bland'. Examples of this spectrum are given for eight different products.

The factors that affect flavour and aroma are discussed and suggestions made as to how the aroma and flavour of different food products might be enhanced. The section closes with a flavour/odour additives chooser chart.

## Designing for colour

The importance of colour is discussed and ways of achieving the desired colour are described – adding coloured ingredients, using food colouring, choice of ingredients and cooking methods. Ways of preventing undesirable colour changes are described and the section closes with a discussion of colour control in industry.

## Designing for texture

This section uses the idea of spectrum of intensity – from 'hard' through 'crisp', 'crunchy', 'crumbly', 'chewy', 'gooey' and 'creamy' eventually to 'soft'. Examples of this spectrum are given for eight different products. The factors that affect texture are discussed and the chapter closes with three chooser charts describing how texture may be modified for main ingredients, flour-based products and sauces.

### Designing for finish

This section describes how important finishing processes – shaping, controlling surface colour, controlling surface texture and adding garnishes – can be used in assembling, cooking and adding finishing touches to food products.

### Designing for the shelf-life of a product

This section begins by describing the importance of shelf-life and summarizing the main means of prolonging it. The section continues by discussing the effects of extending shelf-life on the quality of food materials. It describes the effects of canning, freezing and drying and provides students with guidelines to help them minimize the effects of such processes in the products they design and make.

### Designing for cost

This section begins by discussing the factors that influence the price of a food product, indicating that the greater the amount of processing involved, the greater the price. Ways of keeping costs low in both home cooking and industry are also described.

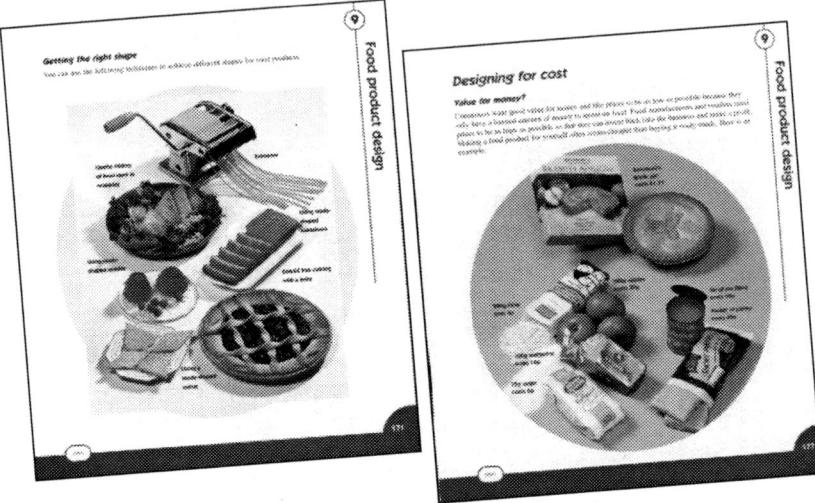

## Chapter 10 Food production

This chapter is divided into three sections.

### Prototype production

This section provides four chooser charts summarizing techniques that are important in making food products – ways to prepare, combine, cook and finish food materials. The aim of the section is to provide students with the information to choose the most appropriate methods for making their food products – usually a single prototype or small batch. Clearly the information will not impart the tacit know-how required to use the methods safely and effectively. There is no substitute for clear skills instruction and the opportunity to practise, so it is important that you use sound demonstration linked to appropriate Resource Tasks to enable students to increase their making skills.

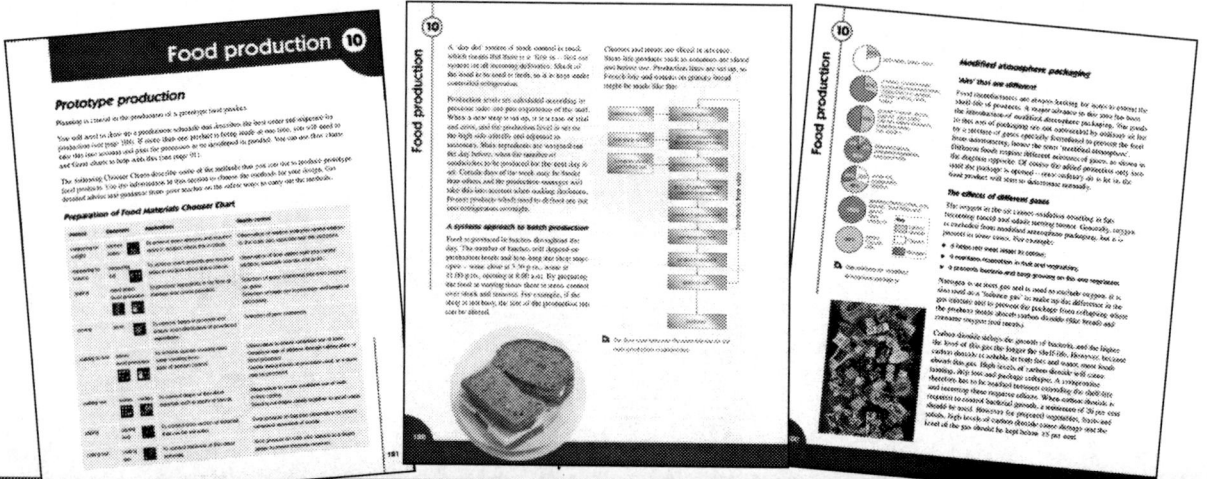

## Catering

This section provides detailed descriptions of the methods used by a chain of sandwich bars and a large hotel. You can use this section to help students appreciate the difference between prototyping and catering and also to plan batch production or catering exercises.

## Industrial production

This section begins by describing the role of control in achieving quality. It discusses the role of sensors and the central processing unit, linking these to the moving of raw materials, mixing ingredients and heating and cooling foods. It describes the difference between quality assurance and quality control and discusses the role of Hazard Analysis and Critical Control Points in the design of manufacturing systems. The section then describes three examples of industrial production – manufacturing jam, frozen vegetables and modified atmosphere packaging.

# Chapter 11 Food sales

This chapter is divided into four sections.

## Food poisoning

This section describes the symptoms and causes of food poisoning, dealing in detail with bacterial contamination and how this can be prevented.

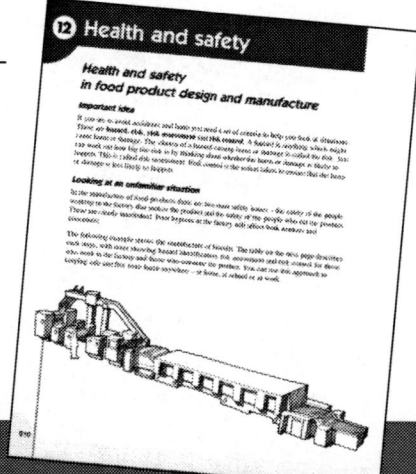

## Food hygiene and the law

This section covers food hygiene legislation and how it operates to prevent food poisoning.

## Food safety and the law

This section covers food safety legislation and how it operates to ensure that food for sale is fit for human consumption.

## Food labelling

This section describes the requirements of the Food Labelling Regulations. It discusses nutritional labelling, permitted food additives and how they affect our food.

# Chapter 12 Health and safety

This chapter revisits the important ideas established earlier – hazards, risks, risk assessment and risk control – and uses them to look at an unfamiliar situation, which is the manufacture of biscuits in a large food factory.

## Specifying a Capability Task

The Nuffield Project has identified the following 15 features that should be explained in order to describe a Capability Task and the associated learning for 14–16 year-olds. It is based on the successful model used earlier, but five of the features are new.

**1 The task** A short statement that indicates the type of product students will design and make.

**2 Task setting** It is important that the task is placed in a setting that can be investigated in a way that informs the subsequent designing and making. The investigation should answer the following questions.

- Who is the product for?

- What is it for?

- Where will it be used?

- When will it be used?

- Is it a one-off or to be mass produced?

- Where might it be sold?

- Who is likely to buy it?

**3 The aims of the task** These will indicate what is to be taught through the task. This will be linked to the type of product the students will design and make and usually include four features:

- learning and using some strategies;

- learning and using some technical knowledge and understanding;

- learning and using some communication techniques;

- learning and using some making skills.

**4 Values** It is important for students to appreciate the values that inform the nature of the need or opportunity and find ways to take them into account. This is more complicated than features 5 and 6 as the detail of the value considerations will depend on the nature of the task setting. This will be revealed by the students' investigations of the setting and for this they will need appropriate strategies. These will be detailed in a programme of study or syllabus and can be taught through an appropriate set or sequence of Resource Tasks (see feature 9).

It will be important for students to consider their own values and move towards a recognition and understanding of the values of others. They will need to think about situations where there are value conflicts and move from simple two-sided arguments to understanding complicated conflicts involving many-sided arguments. Arguments where qualitative values, such as aesthetic considerations, are in conflict with quantitative values, for example, economic considerations, are probably the most difficult to resolve.

The values are presented under the following headings:

- technical  • economic  • aesthetic  • moral  • social  • environmental

They do not represent mutually exclusive sets and there will often be an overlap between the categories. Reading and thinking about Case Studies is a useful way to develop values thinking (see feature 10).

**5  The nature of the product** This has three sections.

'Exploration' lists a selection of written work that should be developed through the initial stages of the task. This always includes a preliminary specification.

'Production and promotion' lists a selection of written work that should be developed to ensure promotion or marketing of the product and quality-assured production. To meet this last feature, a detailed specification is always required, which includes ingredients, equipment and a production schedule.

'Possible products' describes the sort of product the students will design and make at a level of detail that indicates the knowledge, understanding and skills likely to be required to do this. For example, a simple biscuit made from a given recipe, albeit in an interesting shape and well-decorated with icing, requires only basic knowledge, understanding and skill. A filled biscuit product, like a bourbon biscuit, where the top biscuit has been press-moulded, so that there is a raised design with lettering, is a much more complicated product, requiring more detailed knowledge, understanding and skill. There is a dynamic relationship between the nature of the product and the knowledge and understanding of technical matters and making skills. Complicated products *demand* high-level knowledge and skill; high-level knowledge and skill *lead to* complicated products.

**6  Technical knowledge and understanding** This is related to the nature of the product the students are designing and making and can be cross-referenced with the programme of study or syllabus and taught through an appropriate set or sequence of Resource Tasks (see feature 9).

**7  Specialist tools, materials and equipment** For 14–16 year-olds it is assumed that most general-purpose hand tools, light food processing equipment, conventional and microwave ovens and so on will be available. Only specialist or unusual items will be noted. Similarly with ingredients, only the uncommon ones will be detailed.

**8  Cross-curricular links** The use of other areas of knowledge and understanding should be such that they aid the students' designing and making. The approach of, say, science to a particular area – such as polymers – will not necessarily generate understanding that is applicable in a design and technology task. Producing a starch set is a very different task from showing that you can see a light beam pass through a starch sol. However, if the design and technology teacher uses a very different approach, concentrating perhaps on practical application rather than an underlying explanation, this may only serve to confuse the student further. So, it is important to check with colleagues in other curriculum areas and try to use a consistent approach across them all, even though it will be for different purposes.

The cross-curricular links are summarized using headings that indicate a particular subject or theme, such as using art or economic and industrial understanding.

**9  Useful Resource Tasks** A listing of relevant Resource Tasks is always provided. Only you will know which ones are appropriate for your students. Depending on their previous experience and learning, they may need to do all of the suggested tasks, some or only a few. In a very few cases, a student may not need to do any, but this is likely to be a rare exception, as an important feature of capability is the ability to use new knowledge, understanding and skills.

**10 Useful Case Studies** A listing of relevant Case Studies is always provided. However, only you will know which ones are appropriate for your students or how best to use them – with the whole class, with a small group or with an individual. They do provide an important opportunity for the student to reflect on the wider issues of design and technology as well as more focused work concerning quality, products and applications.

A clear description of 1–10 above provides a detailed specification for a Capability Task. This whole approach makes it clear what you have to teach in order that students will become capable in design and technology. It is only when the teaching requirements are clear that you can organize lessons so that learning can take place. However, in order to enable you to modify the tasks and start them at different points from usual (see page 21), the following features are also described.

**11 Design brief** This will always describe the following features:

- the sort of product that is to be made and its purpose;
- who will use it;
- where it will be used;
- where it might be sold.

**12 Preliminary specification** This will always describe the following features:

- what it should do;
- what it should look like;
- other features, such as:
  – how it might be promoted;
  – how it might be eaten;
  – specific consumers groups;
  – particular ingredients to be used;
  – how it should be packaged.

**13 Possible associated activities** This section makes suggestions of activities that do not fall into the Case Study or Resource Task categories that you might wish to include in the task. It is here that opportunities for visits and visiting speakers are noted.

**14 Design sketches** These will give an impression of one or two products that could be made in response to the brief and specification. There will be limited annotation, but insufficient information for the student to make the product without some more design input.

**15 Recipes** These will appear in the text where required and will detail ingredients and amounts and give basic instructions for making, but will not give a detailed production schedule or a detailed sensory specification that the product has to meet. They will deal with simple rather than complicated products. This enables you to shorten the Capability Task considerably and ask students to deal solely with redesign or manufacturing issues.

# How the Capability Tasks are presented

Capability Tasks for 14–16 year-olds are presented as four copymaster A4 overview sheets so that the information is easily and rapidly accessible.

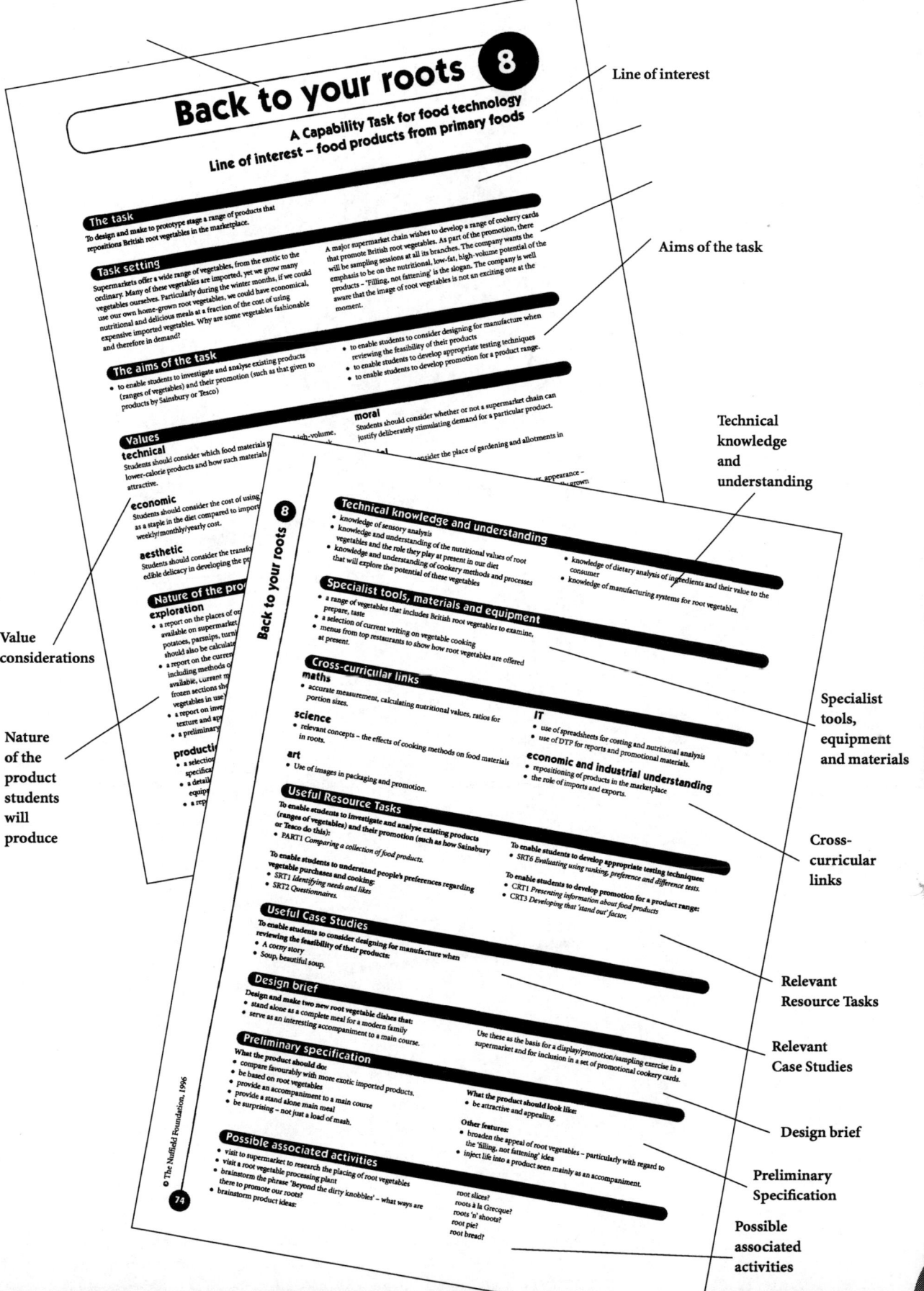

Line of interest

Aims of the task

Technical knowledge and understanding

Value considerations

Nature of the product students will produce

Specialist tools, equipment and materials

Cross-curricular links

Relevant Resource Tasks

Relevant Case Studies

Design brief

Preliminary Specification

Possible associated activities

The detail of the overview sheets:

## Back to your roots 8

A Capability Task for food technology
Line of interest – food products from primary foods

### The task
To design and make to prototype stage a range of products that repositions British root vegetables in the marketplace.

### Task setting
Supermarkets offer a wide range of vegetables, from the exotic to the ordinary. Many of these vegetables are imported, yet we grow many vegetables ourselves. Particularly during the winter months, if we could use our own home-grown root vegetables, we could have economical, nutritional and delicious meals at a fraction of the cost of using expensive imported vegetables. Why are some vegetables fashionable and therefore in demand?

A major supermarket chain wishes to develop a range of cookery cards that promote British root vegetables. As part of the promotion, there will be sampling sessions at all its branches. The company wants the emphasis to be on the nutritional, low-fat, high-volume potential of the products – 'Filling, not fattening' is the slogan. The company is well aware that the image of root vegetables is not an exciting one at the moment.

### The aims of the task
- to enable students to investigate and analyse existing products (ranges of vegetables) and their promotion (such as that given to products by Sainsbury or Tesco)
- to enable students to consider designing for manufacture when reviewing the feasibility of their products
- to enable students to develop appropriate testing techniques
- to enable students to develop promotion for a product range.

### Values
**technical**
Students should consider which food materials [...] lower-calorie products and how such materials [...] attractive.

**economic**
Students should consider the cost of using [...] as a staple in the diet compared to impor[...] weekly/monthly/yearly cost.

**aesthetic**
Students should consider the transfo[...] edible delicacy in developing the pr[...]

**moral**
Students should consider whether or not a supermarket chain can justify deliberately stimulating demand for a particular product.

### Nature of the pro[...]
**exploration**
- a report on the places of o[...] available on supermarket [...] potatoes, parsnips, turni[...] should also be calculate[...]
- a report on the curren[...] including methods o[...] available, current m[...] frozen sections sh[...] vegetables in use [...]
- a report on inve[...] texture and ap[...]
- a preliminary [...]

**producti[...]**
- a selection [...] specificati[...]
- a detail[...] equipm[...]
- a rep[...]

© The Nuffield Foundation, 1996

74

### Technical knowledge and understanding
- knowledge of sensory analysis
- knowledge and understanding of the nutritional values of root vegetables and the role they play at present in our diet
- knowledge and understanding of cookery methods and processes that will explore the potential of these vegetables
- knowledge of dietary analysis of ingredients and their value to the consumer
- knowledge of manufacturing systems for root vegetables.

### Specialist tools, materials and equipment
- a range of vegetables that includes British root vegetables to examine, prepare, taste
- a selection of current writing on vegetable cooking
- menus from top restaurants to show how root vegetables are offered at present.

### Cross-curricular links
**maths**
- accurate measurement, calculating nutritional values, ratios for portion sizes.

**science**
- relevant concepts – the effects of cooking methods on food materials in roots.

**art**
- Use of images in packaging and promotion.

**IT**
- use of spreadsheets for costing and nutritional analysis
- use of DTP for reports and promotional materials.

**economic and industrial understanding**
- repositioning of products in the marketplace
- the role of imports and exports.

### Useful Resource Tasks
To enable students to investigate and analyse existing products (ranges of vegetables) and their promotion (such as how Sainsbury or Tesco do this):
- PART1 Comparing a collection of food products.

To enable students to understand people's preferences regarding vegetable purchases and cooking:
- SRT1 Identifying needs and likes
- SRT2 Questionnaires.

To enable students to develop appropriate testing techniques:
- SRT6 Evaluating using ranking, preference and difference tests.

To enable students to develop promotion for a product range:
- CRT1 Presenting information about food products
- CRT3 Developing that 'stand out' factor.

### Useful Case Studies
To enable students to consider designing for manufacture when reviewing the feasibility of their products:
- A corny story
- Soup, beautiful soup.

### Design brief
Design and make two new root vegetable dishes that:
- stand alone as a complete meal for a modern family
- serve as an interesting accompaniment to a main course.

Use these as the basis for a display/promotion/sampling exercise in a supermarket and for inclusion in a set of promotional cookery cards.

### Preliminary specification
**What the product should do:**
- compare favourably with more exotic imported products
- be based on root vegetables
- provide an accompaniment to a main course
- provide a stand alone main meal
- be surprising – not just a load of mash.

**What the product should look like:**
- be attractive and appealing.

**Other features:**
- broaden the appeal of root vegetables – particularly with regard to the 'filling, not fattening' idea
- inject life into a product seen mainly as an accompaniment.

### Possible associated activities
- visit to supermarket to research the placing of root vegetables
- visit a root vegetable processing plant
- brainstorm the phrase 'Beyond the dirty knobbles' – what ways are there to promote our roots?
- brainstorm product ideas:

root slices?
roots à la Grecque?
roots 'n' shoots?
root pie?
root bread?

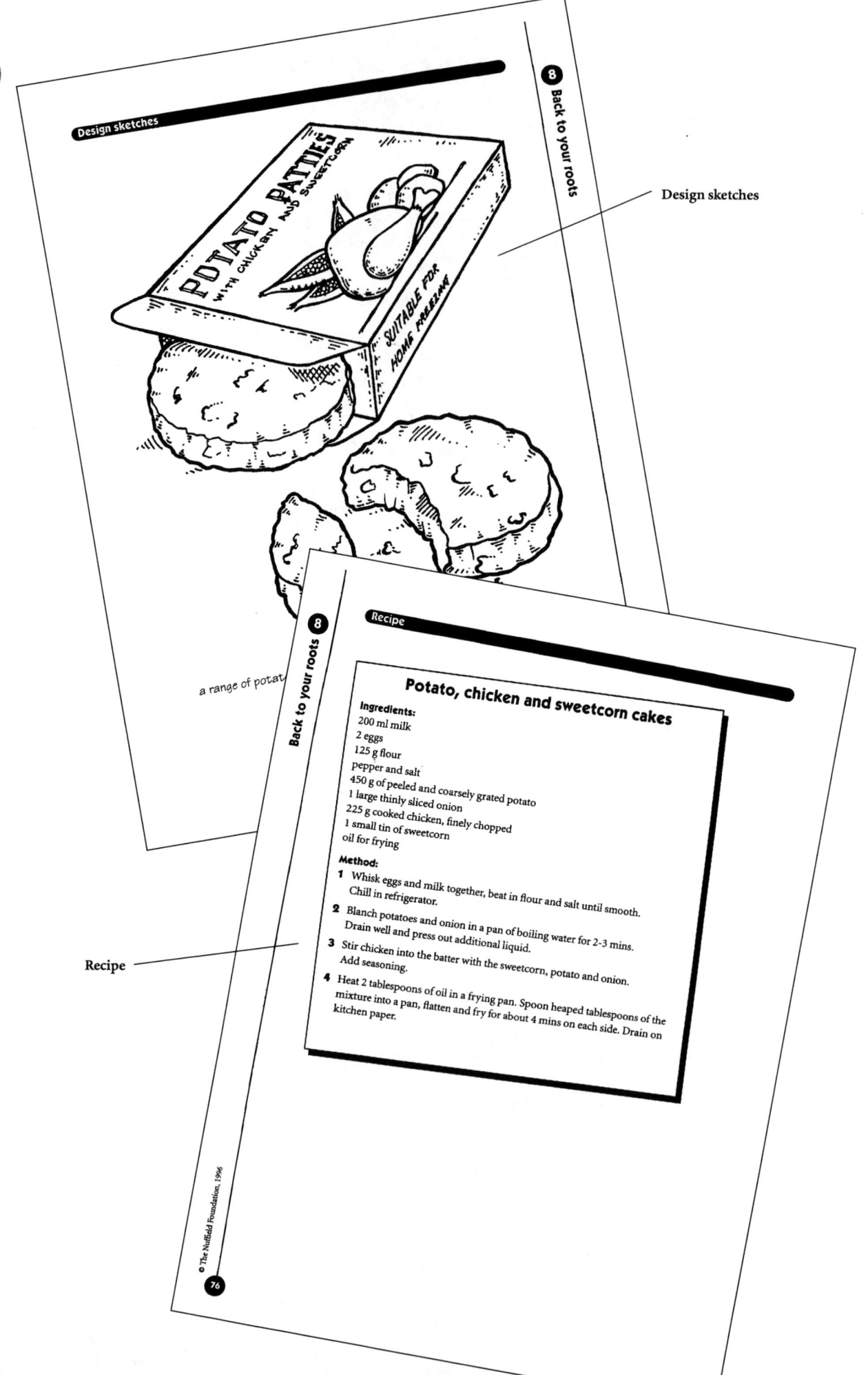

**Design sketches**

POTATO PATTIES
WITH CHICKEN AND SWEETCORN

SUITABLE FOR HOME FREEZING

Design sketches

a range of potat

**Recipe**

### Potato, chicken and sweetcorn cakes

**Ingredients:**
200 ml milk
2 eggs
125 g flour
pepper and salt
450 g of peeled and coarsely grated potato
1 large thinly sliced onion
225 g cooked chicken, finely chopped
1 small tin of sweetcorn
oil for frying

**Method:**
1 Whisk eggs and milk together, beat in flour and salt until smooth. Chill in refrigerator.

2 Blanch potatoes and onion in a pan of boiling water for 2-3 mins. Drain well and press out additional liquid.

3 Stir chicken into the batter with the sweetcorn, potato and onion. Add seasoning.

4 Heat 2 tablespoons of oil in a frying pan. Spoon heaped tablespoons of the mixture into a pan, flatten and fry for about 4 mins on each side. Drain on kitchen paper.

Recipe

76

# Using the Capability Tasks to plan a full GCSE course

## Managing three Capability Tasks

It is likely that your students will tackle three Capability Tasks during year 10, each one from a different line of interest. You can work out which ones your class will tackle. In year 11, students can revisit a line of interest or tackle a new one. The task worked on in year 11 will probably be the one that is used for their GCSE course work. This makes sense because the students should be better at designing and making in year 11 than they were in year 10. It will be quite a struggle to fit three complete Capability Tasks into year 10 so you may wish to organize the lessons so that students only do part of some of these tasks. They will certainly need to do one complete Capability Task where they design, make and test a well-finished product. There are several ways to shorten Capability Tasks.

- You might shorten it so that the students produce a prototype product without refining it to develop improved versions. This means that the time spent is reduced as the students don't have to spend a lot of time improving their food product.

- You might decide that the students should only produce a series of design proposals or recipe suggestions as detailed annotated sketches. This cuts down the time they spend on the Capability Task even further.

- You may decide to give the class a design brief plus a preliminary specification and ask them to develop a detailed specification from which to design and make a product. This removes all of the task-setting investigation from the task, plus brief and preliminary specification development, and so lessens the time spent.

- You could decide to give the class the brief, specification and some design sketches as a starting point. This will cut down the design development phase even further.

- You might even give the class the brief, the preliminary specification and a recipe and ask them to make the product because, for example, they need to concentrate on manufacturing or redesign issues. This will reduce the time spent even further.

Example briefs, specifications, design sketches and recipes are included in the Capability Tasks so that you have control over the time spent on the tasks. Of course, it is important that the students still carry out the Resource Tasks and Case Studies needed for each of the Capability Tasks. In this way, they can learn lots of design and technology knowledge, understanding and skill and still keep in touch with designing and making. This will put the students in a strong position to tackle a full Capability Task in year 11. It is important that the students know at the outset of the Capability Task how long it is going to take and in what way it will be shortened from being a full Capability Task. They need to be quite clear as to the expected outcomes. There is little that is more disappointing for a student than to start a Capability Task with the expectation of taking home a finished piece only to be told during the task 'Well, we haven't got time to finish so a recipe suggestion will do'.

### Short course requirements

If you are teaching a short course, you will need to reduce the number of Capability Tasks accordingly and perhaps complete just one full and one reduced-time task before students tackle their main task for GCSE assessment.

## ⑤ Choosing the lines of interest

The lines of interest have been chosen because they represent different degrees of risk as far as the teacher is concerned. Some of the lines of interest involve students designing and making products with which most teachers are quite familiar and the likelihood of the students being successful is high. This is simply because the teacher is so familiar with the knowledge, understanding and skill required for success and the typical pitfalls that he or she can teach appropriately to the task and provide effective guidance without the student losing ownership of the work. Other lines of interest are slightly less safe and the majority of teachers may feel some concern about the level of success they can guarantee with students designing and making these sorts of products. Some other lines of interest may be seen as high-risk ones in that they are outside the previous experience of the teacher. Exactly what constitutes a risk to you and the level of that risk will depend on your specialist training, any in-service training you may have received, the facilities in your school and your previous teaching experience. So, while only you can make the best judgement, the Nuffield Project does offer this guidance. Of the three Capability Tasks you might teach in year 10, choose two that are low-risk ones. In this way, the bulk of your work in year 10 is likely to be successful. If, for some reason, you are not successful in this area of risk, then the damage is easy to limit. If, however, you are successful, this is good professional development and, over a period of time, this part of your teaching will cease to be one of risk and become an area of guaranteed success. You will then be in a position to tackle a further and different area of risk in the knowledge that you can be successful.

## In-built assessment through reviewing

It is important that your students work in a way that reveals their design and technology thinking. Evidence of their capability should emerge quite naturally from the way they tackle a Capability Task. The way students review the progress of their work during a Capability Task is an important means of providing you with assessment evidence. From the students' viewpoint, reviewing is essential for two reasons. First, it demands that students stop and reflect on what they have done so far and the consequences of this for further action. Thus, it is an important strategy in giving students a sense that designing is a coherent and continuous activity; that the activity is not a series of unconnected steps prompted, perhaps, by teacher intervention or worksheet instruction. It is important for the student to view designing as a sequence of connected activities over which they have some control. Reviewing helps to establish this view. Second, in confronting students with the consequences of their actions, the review procedure can provide momentum for the task in that it forces students to make decisions about what to do next.

In one sense, reviewing should be happening continuously as every action should be the result of a plan–execute–review cycle.

- 'I plan to take a particular course of action because …'
- 'I do it'
- 'I reflect on the result of the doing (that is, I review the consequences of my actions) and use these thoughts to plan my next action and so on.'

It is quite impossible to monitor this continuous and ongoing reviewing within a student's work, but the Nuffield Project has identified the following three staging posts in design activity where a more formal review is extremely useful.

### First review

Once students have some ideas for their products in the form of quickly drawn annotated sketches, they should carry out their first review by comparing their ideas with the requirements of the brief and the specification. They should ask themselves the following questions for each design idea.

- Will the design do what it is supposed to?
- Will the design be suitable for the users?
- Will the design fit in with where it might be used or sold?
- Is the design likely to work?
- Does the design look right for the users and sellers?
- Have I noted any special requirements the design will need to meet later on?

Any design ideas that do not get a 'yes' for all these questions will need to be rejected or adjusted. In this way, they can use the first review to screen out any design ideas that will not meet their requirements. They can do this screening in two ways:

- as an individual, by just sitting, thinking it through in their heads and making notes against each design idea;
- they can work in a group and explain their ideas to other students who can check them out against the questions.

This latter method takes longer and each student has to help the others in the group check out their design ideas, but the extra time involved is usually well spent as the overall level of constructive criticism is higher.

Whichever method you choose for your students to review their work, it is important that they discuss their review findings with you.

## Second review

By screening their early ideas, students will be able to focus their efforts on developing a completed food product. It is important to produce a first prototype quickly so that they can test it and modify it in a series of second-stage reviews. They should record the story of these modifications as a mixture of annotated sketches describing the effects of changes in cooking methods, ingredients, freezing and thawing, the results of tasting sessions, photographs, sometimes rendered presentation drawings and the instructions for making the recipes and so on.

To make sure that they follow a sensible direction for developing their product, they will need to ask the following questions as they test and modify it.

- Does it meet the flavour and texture requirements?
- Is the appearance (shape, size, colour) suitable?
- Does it meet nutritional requirements?
- Can I purchase the ingredients within the agreed budget?
- Will it have the required storage characteristics?

Once they are satisfied that their product will meet the requirements of the specification, they can produce a final version. They will need to be clear about the time available for this final making and ask themselves the following questions.

- Will the ingredients I need be available when I need them?
- Will the tools and equipment be available when I need them?
- Am I sure that I can get the final appearance that I need?
- Have I got enough time for finishing and presenting my food product?
- Is there anything I can do to make producing the product more efficient?

The individual student is probably the only one who can answer these questions, but it is important that you establish the routine where they check their answers with you in order to avoid hidden traps and pitfalls.

## Third review

Once the design has been produced, students should review their products to check how the products perform against their specifications, attribute profiles, user reactions, winner/loser balance and appropriateness. There are Resource Tasks that revise these methods of evaluation and it is important to make these product evaluation sessions active. One way to do this is for you to organize students into discussion groups. Each student gives their product a blob score for each part of the specification – five blobs if it meets that part really well, three blobs if it meets it moderately well, one blob if it meets it only poorly and no blobs if it fails to meet this part of the specification. Each student, in turn, then explains to the other students in the group why these scores have been given. The rest of the group question these judgements. Each student has to convince the others that the judgements are correct. This activity is a powerful precursor to looking at overall progress.

## Students looking at their own progress

At the end of a Capability Task, it is important for students to look back at what they have done and reflect on their progress. The *Student's Book* contains the following sets of questions to help students do this.

### Feeling good about what you have done

- Am I proud of what I have made?
- Can I explain why?
- Am I proud of the design I developed?
- Can I explain why?

### Understanding the problems

- What sorts of things slowed me down?
- Can I now see how to overcome these sorts of difficulties?
- What sorts of things made me nervous so that I didn't do as well as I know I can?
- Do I know where to get help now?
- What sort of things did I do better than I expected?
- Was this due to luck or can I say that I'm getting better?
- Were there times when I concentrated on detail before I had the broad picture?
- Were there times when I didn't bother enough with detail?
- Can I now see how to get the level of detail right?

### Understanding yourself

- Were there times when I lost interest?
- Can I now see how to get myself motivated?
- Were there times when I couldn't work out what to do next?
- Can I now see how to get better at making decisions?
- Were there times when I lost my sense of direction?
- Can I now see how to avoid this?

### Understanding my design decisions

- With hindsight, can I see where I made the right decisions?
- With hindsight, can I see where I should have made different decisions?
- With hindsight, can I see situations where I did the right thing?
- With hindsight, can I see where I would do things differently if I did this again?

You can use students' answers to these questions to see strengths and weaknesses and to identify areas for improvement.

## Examination questions

The Nuffield Project has identified eight types of questions that may be set for GCSE written, terminal examinations. It is important that you are familiar with these and teach your students to respond appropriately to each type .

## Type 1: knowledge definitions

The candidate is expected to show understanding of key terms, principles and concepts. The question will be written in a form that requires candidates to *recognize* or *give an example* that illustrates the meaning, but candidates will not be expected to be able to recall and state a definition.

### Example

A local café called Coffee Time has asked you to design a new logo to use on their menu. They want the logo to *appeal* to their customers.

**For recognition**

Imagine you are writing a questionnaire to check which of your two logo designs is most *appealing*, which of the following questions would you include?

- Which logo looks most interesting?
- Which logo would Coffee Time like best?
- Which logo would make you want to buy a coffee?
- Which logo do you like?

**For giving examples**

Imagine you need to write a questionnaire to check which of your two logo designs is most *appealing*. Suggest three suitable questions.

Both of these aspects could be extended to ask students to *explain* their choices and describe *methods* for carrying out the survey and collecting and presenting results.

## Type 2: knowledge of purpose ('Why?')

The candidate is expected to show understanding of:

- why things are done in a particular way ('Why do it in that way?');
- why actions or decisions are significant or important ('Why would you do x?' or 'Why is it like that?');
- why decisions are appropriate or have been made ('Why has it been made from x?').

The question will be written in such a way that the student has to explain or justify something.

### Example

The candidate will be given information about a product in the form of annotated illustrations and text. They will be asked to explain different features of the design, such as:

- why a particular ingredient has been chosen;
- why a part is the shape and form that it is.

This could be extended to ask students to explain the *method* they used or *predict* the effects of changed variables or make a *creative response*.

## Type 3: knowledge of method ('How?')

The candidate is expected to describe or explain, showing an understanding of:

- processes, materials and techniques ('How could I make this design from particular materials?');
- the application of technological principles ('Show how you would do x or make x happen');
- the application of design strategies ('How would you research, analyse, review, make decisions, plan, test, evaluate and so on?').

The question will be written in a form that asks students to *describe* using a suitable mode of response, such as notes and diagrams, grid/matrix, flow chart and so on.

### Example

The candidate will be given information about a product in the form of annotated illustrations and text and asked:

- how a particular ingredient might be prepared;
- how risks can be avoided when using a necessary technique;
- how a product could be adapted to make it cost less;
- how a product could be adapted to make it less fattening;
- how a product might be packaged;
- how to carry out a user trip;
- how to calculate costs of making.

## Type 4: speculating about change ('What if?')

The candidate will be asked to predict the results of given changes in circumstances or variables, including:
- the direct consequences of things ('What would happen if you did x?');
- the effect on connected things ('If you changed x then what effect would this have on y?').

The question will be written in a form that asks the student to *suggest what would happen if*.

### Example

The candidate will be presented with a recipe using self-raising flour and asked the following.
- What would happen if you used plain flour?
- If you only had plain flour, what could you do to create the effect of using self-raising flour?
- What effect would this have on the resulting food product?
- What could you do to alleviate this effect?

## Type 5: creative problem solving

The candidate will be asked to develop a *personal response* to a short technical design problem. The question will be written in a form that requires students to *suggest* possible solutions, *compare* their alternatives and select and *justify a recommended* solution.

### Example

The candidate will be presented with an incomplete design to which there are several different possible solutions. Three things might then be asked of them, such as:
- use notes and sketches to illustrate two possible solutions to the problem;
- make a list for each of your ideas to show the strengths and weaknesses of your solutions;
- state clearly which idea you think is the best and give your reasons.

It is here that some formal requirements to use mathematics or science can be included in the question.

## Type 6: design strategies

The candidate will be asked to use design *strategies* for a short design scenario. The question will be written in a form that requires the student to *use a given strategy* to carry out design analysis, development or evaluation.

Strategies could include:
- clarifying briefs – turning an open-ended brief into a more specific form;
- writing specifications – turning a headline specification into a more detailed form;
- attribute analysis – analysing possible product characteristics;
- brainstorming – completing a started brainstorm or organizing a random list from a brainstorm to show categories and links;
- impact of D&T – interrogating a completed winners and losers chart;
- user trip – interpreting user views and opinions.

### Example

The candidate will be presented with a series of images showing the reactions of someone eating or using a product. For example a taste testing – image 1, smelling; image 2, tasting; image 3, looking; image 4, touching/cutting/breaking/ and so on.

The candidate will be told that these photos were taken of someone testing a new food product that was designed to … (simple brief).

The candidate will be asked to:
- write down what they think the person was asked to do
- how they think this person responded to the product
- write down the reactions of the person tasting the product.

## Type 7: presenting and interpreting information

The candidate will be asked to make sense of D&T research data.
> The question will be written in a form which requires a student to:
- *present* the information clearly;
- *interpret* the data and reach conclusions.

### Example

The candidate will be given data from some design and technology research that may come from very different sources. It could be about:
- consumer preferences;
- the results of testing a material or component;
- sales figures for different products.

**To present**
- Draw a graph or chart to show what people of different age groups thought about the old version of the soft drink as compared with the new version.
- Think carefully about which would be the most appropriate form of graph or chart to use to present the data clearly.

**To interpret**
- Which age group of consumers has changed its views most about soft drinks?
- Write down which you think it is and give reasons for your view.

## Type 8: interpreting a short Case Study

The candidate will be asked to use *comprehension* skills, design *strategies* and *knowledge* to demonstrate their *understanding* of D&T activity from the world outside school. The question will be written in a form that requires the student to:
- *find* a piece of *information* from the text
- *explain* something that is described in the text
- *make judgements* about the quality and effects of the design and technology described.
    It is here also that the application of science or mathematics may be built into the question.

### Example

The case study could describe how packaging has changed over the last 50 years and a short piece about modified atmosphere packaging. The candidate could be asked to:
**Find information**
- How were eggs and biscuits packaged in 1950?
- How are eggs and biscuits packaged now?

**Explain**
- Explain why it is important for the packaging for eggs to be rigid.
- Explain what happens to the shelf-life of a product when modified atmosphere packaging is opened to the ordinary atmosphere.

**Make judgements**
- Explain why some pressure groups are campaigning for the use of less packaging.
- Explain why some food manufacturers use packaging to provide nutritional information not required by law.

This chapter provides a brief summary of the requirements of different Examination Boards and indicates those syllabuses that are supported by Nuffield materials.

## City and Guilds of London Institute

**City&
Guilds**

### Courses being offered

The following are being offered as both full and short GCSE courses:
Design and Technology (unendorsed – two focus areas)
Design and Technology: Resistant Materials Technology[†]
Design and Technology: Food Technology[†]
Design and Technology: Textile Technology[†]
Design and Technology: Graphic Products[†]
Design and Technology: Electronic Products[†].
A combined course in Design and technology and Business Enterprise will also be offered.
[†]Are supported by Nuffield materials.

### Coursework requirements

This is in two parts.

- Candidates are required to produce an integrated design and make the project duration approximately 20 hours for a short course or 40 hours for a full course.

- Candidates are required to produce a written product evaluation report on an existing product.

Course work accounts for 60 per cent of the total marks (one third for designing, two thirds for making) and will be moderated by external moderators visiting the centre.

### Examination requirements

For the short course, candidates are required to take a one hour and 25-minute examination based on section A of the syllabus.

For the full course, candidates are required to take the same one hour and 25-minute examination as the short course candidates, plus a further paper of one hour and 25 minutes based on section B of the syllabus.

The examination counts for 40 per cent of the total marks (50 per cent designing, 50 per cent making). There are two tiers for written papers: A*–D and C–G.

### Key features

- Allows candidates to specialize in a single materials focus area or work in two focus areas.

- Provides a teacher support guide.

- Links with GNVQs at Foundation and Intermediate levels.

- Detailed assessment course work grid with criteria for each GCSE grade.

- External moderator support.

- Specified requirements of design applications in an industrial context.

- Prepares students for the technological world, requiring them to design and make products in response to needs and opportunities.

**For further information contact:**
Subject Officer  Tel: 0171 294 2468  Fax: 0171 294 2400

## ⑦ Midland Examining Group

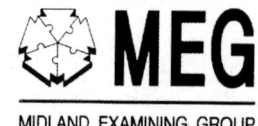

### Courses being offered

The following are being offered as both full and short GCSE courses:

D&T: Resistant Materials Technology†

D&T: Textile Technology†

D&T: Graphic Products†

D&T: Electronic Products†.

D&T: Food Technology†

The following are being offered as full GCSE courses only:

D&T: Systems and Control Products

D&T: Automotive Engineering

D&T Engineering (both full and dual award).

†Are supported by Nuffield materials.

### Course work requirements

All course work has an overall weighting of 60 per cent.

For syllabuses offered as both full and short GCSE courses, candidates are required to complete a course work project – a design folder and realization of a quality product. For the full course, this represents 40 to 60 hours of curriculum time, for the short course, 20 to 30 hours.

For D&T Systems and Control Products, candidates are required to complete a course work project – a design folder and realization of a system/control product.

For D&T Automotive Engineering, candidates are required to complete a course work project – a design folder and the realization of a system/control product (40 per cent) and practical assignments (20 per cent).

For D&T Engineering, candidates are required to produce a portfolio selection of work. In addition, dual award candidates will have to complete a response to an engineering design brief and an engineering report.

### Examination requirements

All terminal examinations have an overall weighting of 40 per cent. There are two tiers of entry: higher – A\* to D (U) and foundation – C to G.

For the syllabuses being offered as both full and short GCSE courses, candidates taking a short course take one paper, while candidates taking a full course take two papers.

For D&T: Systems and Control Products, candidates take two papers – paper 1, core, and paper 2, option.

For D&T: Automotive Engineering, candidates take one paper.

For D&T: Engineering, candidates complete a Board-set Capability Task (duration ten hours) and take one paper for the single award or two papers for the dual award.

#### Key features

- All assessments are weighted: designing 40 per cent, making 60 per cent.
- Schools and candidates can choose from a wide range of D&T focus areas.
- All course work is internally assessed and standardized; moderation will be by visit.
- Allow candidates to produce a realistic product for course work.
- New, 'user-friendly' course work assessment scheme.
- Full INSET programme commenced October 1995.

#### For further information contact:

Subject Officer  Tel: 0115 929 6021  Fax: 0115 929 5261

# Northern Examinations and Assessment Board

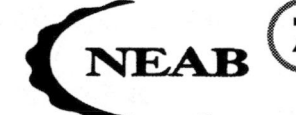

## Courses being offered

The following are being offered as both full and short GCSE courses:
Design and Technology: Resistant Materials†
Design and Technology: Graphic Products†
Design and Technology: Food Technology†
Design and Technology: Textile Technology†
Design and Technology: Electronic Products†

The following is being offered as a full GCSE course only:
Design and Technology: Systems.
†Are supported by Nuffield materials.

## Course work requirements

Course work submission is 60 per cent of the overall assessment (20 per cent designing and 40 per cent making).

Candidates are required to complete a major project consisting of a design folder and a practical outcome. The project will be assessed holistically using the two assessment objectives, 'designing and making'.

The time to be spent on the project will depend on the material area. The short course requirements are half those for the full course, so Design and Technology: Resistant Materials is about 50/25 hours and Design and Technology: Food Technology, 25/12 hours.

## Examination requirements

Examinations count for 40 per cent of the total marks.

All candidates sit a single written paper, set at two tiers, with separate papers for the full and short courses.

For the full course, higher-level candidates (Grades A*–D), take a written paper of two and a half hours and foundation-level candidates (Grades C–G) take a two-hour written paper.

For the short course, higher-level candidates (Grades A*–D) take a written paper for two hours and foundation-level candidates (Grades C–G) take a one and a half-hour written paper.

## Key features

- All syllabuses build on the good practice developed in the current Design and Technology and Technology syllabuses.

- Each syllabus may be delivered by an individual teacher.

- A wide range of materials may be used in the Design and Technology Resistant Materials syllabus.

- Common syllabus section based on the Design and Technology Programme of Study for designing and making for 14–16 year-olds.

- Moderation is by inspection, normally by visiting moderators.

**For further information contact:**
Subject Officer  Tel: 0191 201 0180  Fax: 0191 271 3314

## ⑦ RSA Examinations Board

### Courses being offered

The following are being offered as both full and short GCSE courses:

Design and Technology (unendorsed, multi-material, covering Resistant Materials)[†]
Design and Technology: Textiles Technology[†]
Design and Technology: Food Technology[†]
Design and Technology: Graphical Products[†]

[†]Are supported by Nuffield materials.

### Course work requirements

Course work accounts for 60 per cent of the total marks (one third for designing, two thirds for making) and will be moderated by externally appointed moderators visiting the centre.

Candidates are required to produce a portfolio of work, including a substantial designing and making task. The substantial task should take approximately 20 hours for the short course and approximately 40 hours for the full course.

### Examination requirements

Examination results count for 40 per cent of the total marks, divided equally between designing and making.

For the short course, candidates are required to take a one-hour examination based on a scenario set by RSA in advance of the examination that draws on the knowledge, skills and understanding identified for the GCSE (short course), including the chosen manufacturing material area.

For the full course, in addition to taking the same one-hour examination as those on the short course, candidates will take a further one-hour extension paper, to show a more detailed knowledge and understanding of working with a design specification in the industrial manufacturing material area they have chosen.

### Key features

- Allows candidates to specialize in a single material or work in more than one material.

- Provides full teacher support, including a support pack and INSET.

- Allows credit towards GNVQ Intermediate Manufacturing Units.

**For further information contact:**
Subject Officer  Tel: 01203 470033  Fax: 01203 468080

# Southern Examining Group

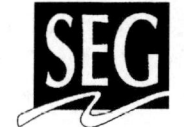

## Courses being offered

Both full and short courses are offered.

The Design and Technology full course syllabus (3400) consists of two parts: 1) a common syllabus section and 2) an area of focus.

Candidates choose from one of the following areas of focus:

Electronic Products[†]

Graphic Products[†]

Systems and Control Products[†]

Product Design and Manufacture[†]

Food Technology[†]

Textile Technology[†]

The Design and Technology short course (1400) consists of the common syllabus section only, without the areas of focus.

[†]Are supported by Nuffield materials.

## Course work requirements

Course work submission makes up 60 per cent of the overall assessment (40 per cent of this being for designing skills, 60 per cent for making skills).

Candidates are required to submit an assignment integrating designing and making supported by additional tasks or, alternatively, two integrated assignments.

Course work submission may be achieved through the common syllabus content and one area of focus.

Moderation will be by area moderation meetings under the direction of an SEG moderator.

## Examination requirements

The written papers of the examination are 40 per cent of the overall assessment (40 per cent for designing and 60 per cent for making).

For the full course, candidates are required to take a written paper of one and a half hours on the common syllabus section and a written paper of one hour on their chosen area of focus.

For the short course, candidates are required to take a written paper of one and a half hours on the common syllabus section.

## Key features

- Common syllabus section based on the Programme of Study for Design and Technology for 14–16 year-olds.

- Builds on the Programme of Study for Design and Technology for 11–14 year-olds.

- Allows centres a flexible approach to the subject.

- Provides specimen question papers and marking schemes.

- Provides a comprehensive teacher support package, including printed exemplar materials, regional support meetings and experienced staff to deal with queries.

## For further information contact:

Subject Officer  Tel: 01483 506506  Fax: 01483 300152

(7) # University of London Examinations & Assessment Council

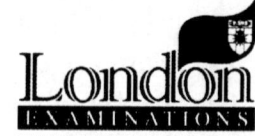

## The following are being offered as both full and short GCSE courses:

Design and Technology: Product Design[†]
Design and Technology: Graphic Products[†]
Design and Technology: Electronic Products[†]
Design and Technology: Food Technology[†]
Design and Technology: Textile Technology[†]

The following combined course is being offered:
Design and Technology: Product Design and Business.
[†]Are supported by Nuffield materials.

## Course work requirements

Course work accounts for 60 per cent of the total marks for both full and short courses.

For the full course, candidates will have to produce one major Capability Task (40 per cent), taking approximately 30 hours, and an assignment (20 per cent), taking approximately 10 hours.

For the short course, candidates will have to produce one major Capability Task (40 per cent), taking approximately 15 hours, and an assignment (20 per cent), taking approximately 5 hours.

Themes for the tasks will be chosen by candidates and approved by teachers in accordance with their chosen focus area and lines of interest. ULEAC will provide exemplar material to guide teachers in selecting and setting tasks.

## Examination requirements

The written papers of the examination are 40 per cent of the overall assessment.
The full course examination lasts two and a half hours.
The short course examination lasts one a half hours.

## Key features

- Each syllabus has a single focus area, which allows candidates to develop their skills in designing and making as well as their knowledge and understanding of a field of special interest to them.

- The skills, knowledge and understanding covered in this syllabus may be realized in a variety of ways, according to the resources available and the interests of teacher and candidates.

- The Council will provide teacher support and guidance for the course work and for the syllabus.

### For further information contact:

Subject Officer  Tel: 0171 331 4000  Fax: 0171 753 4558

# Welsh Joint Education Committee

## Courses being offered

Design and technology is being offered as full, combined and short GCSE courses in the five combined syllabuses. Design and technology may be taken with either art, business studies, catering, electronics or information technology.

All courses may be delivered through one or more of the following six focus areas:

| | |
|---|---|
| Control | Product Design[†] |
| Food[†] | Resistant Materials[†] |
| Graphic Media[†] | Textiles[†]. |

[†]Are supported by Nuffield materials

## Course work requirements

Course work submission is 60 per cent of the overall assessment and there is a 40 : 60 weighting for designing and making.

For a full course, candidates are required to complete a single substantial design and make project, which may be based on one or more of the focus areas.

For a short course, candidates are required to complete a single substantial design and make project, which may be based on one or more of the focus areas, but the depth of study and time commitment of the project is reduced compared to the full course.

Project work will be assessed by the centre and a sample moderated by a visiting examiner.

## Examination requirements and weightings

The written papers of the examination count for 40 per cent of the overall assessment.

For the full course, there will be a terminal examination consisting of two papers, totalling two and a half hours:

- paper 1 is common to all focus areas

- paper 2 is specific to a single focus area – candidates select one from six.

Candidates will be required to demonstrate designing skills and an understanding of making skills applicable to at least one of the focus areas.

For short and combined courses, candidates sit only the first paper.

## Key features

- There are two tiers of entry:
  - Foundation (grades G to C)
  - Higher (grades D to A*).

- Develops candidates' competence to address a wide variety of design situations by drawing on a broad base of knowledge and skills.

- The syllabus provides the opportunity for a number of existing curriculum areas to make a contribution to the examination.

- The syllabus is sufficiently broad, balanced and relevant to interest all candidates.

### For further information contact:

Subject Officer  Tel: 01222 265000  Fax: 01222 575994

| Task number and title | Learning | Type of task | Links with other subjects | Time | Demand | Capability Tasks supported |
|---|---|---|---|---|---|---|
| SRT 1 Identifying needs and likes | To identify needs and likes | Recap | | Part 1: 40 minutes Part 2: 40 minutes | * | Air travel special diets, Weight watchers, Young eaters, Frozen deliveries, Student snack, Soup kitchen, Back to your roots, Luxury cakes, Confectionery by post |
| SRT 2 Questioning | How to make use of information collected in a survey. How to use a database to handle the information. | New | IT | 120 minutes | *** | Air travel special diets, Student snack, Better than a sandwich, Back to your roots, Luxury cakes, Confectionery by post |
| SRT 3 Design briefs and specifications | To extend your understanding of how to write design briefs in response to needs, wants and likes (Part 1) and write a specification from a design brief (Part 2). | Extension | | Part 1: 40 minutes Part 2: 40 minutes | ** | Air travel special diets |
| SRT 4 Brainstorming | To apply two sorts of brainstorming | Extension | | Part 1: 40 minutes Part 2: 40 minutes | ** | Weight watchers, Young eaters, Frozen deliveries, New breads, Better than a sandwich |
| SRT 5 Attribute analysis | To extend your understanding of how to use attribute analysis to think up different ideas for a food product. | Extension | | 45 minutes | ** | Weight watchers, New breads |
| SRT 6 Evaluating 1, Ranking, preference and difference tests | To extend your understanding of using sensory testing to evaluate the acceptability of modified recipes and to use this information to analyse and modify prototype food product. | Extension | | Part 1: 60 minutes Part 2: 20 minutes | * | New breads, Better than a sandwich, Back to your roots |
| SRT 7 Evaluating 2, Winners and losers and appropriateness | To extend your understanding of how to evaluate a product by thinking how it affects people and whether it is appropriate. | Extension | | Part 1: 40 minutes Part 2: 40 minutes | ** | Soup kitchen, Luxury cakes, Confectionery by post |
| SRT 8 Evaluating 3, User trip and performance specification | More about user trips and performance specifications for evaluation. | Extension | | Part 1: 30 minutes Part 2: 30 minutes | ** | Young eaters, Frozen deliveries, New breads, Better than a sandwich, Luxury cakes, Confectionery by post |
| SRT 9 Evaluation by attribute profile | To apply attribute analysis. | New | | Part 1: 40 minutes Part 2: 40 minutes | *** | Soup kitchen, New breads, Better than a sandwich |

# Resource Task Summary Tables

| Task number and title | Learning | Type of task | Links with other subjects | Time | Demand | Capability Tasks supported |
|---|---|---|---|---|---|---|
| CRT 1 Presenting information about food products | To present market research data so that it is attractive and easy to understand. | Extension | IT | 60 minutes | ** | Air travel special diets, Weight watchers, Young eaters, Frozen deliveries, Student snack, Long live fruit, Back to your roots, New breads, Better than a sandwich, Luxury cakes, Confectionery by post |
| CRT 2 Exploring packaging | To understand the role of packaging for food products. | New | | Part 1: 40 minutes Part 2: 30 minutes | ** | Weight watchers, Young eaters, Frozen deliveries, Soup kitchen |
| CRT 3 Develop that stand-out factor | To understand how food product labels can be designed to be appealing, easily identifiable and distinctive. | New | IT, Art | 40 minutes | * | Weight watchers, Young eaters, Frozen deliveries, Long live fruit, Back to your roots |
| CRT 4 Communicating production methods | How to produce a production schedule. | New | | 40 minutes | * | Air travel special diets |
| FCRT 1 Food tests | How to carry out simple food tests for a range of nutrients. Safety note: you should carry these out in a science area, NOT a food preparation area. | New | Science | 120 minutes unless students share results | ** | Can be useful to support a variety of tasks |
| FCRT 2 Making things set | How to control the stiffness of gels using starch. | Extension | Science | Part 1: 60 minutes Part 2: 60 minutes Part 3: 60 minutes | ** | Student snack |
| FCRT 3 Looking at foams | How to control the stability of egg white foams. | New | | 60 minutes | ** | Confectionery by post |
| FCRT 4 Looking at emulsions | How to produce a stable emulsion. | New | Science | 30 minutes | ** | Confectionery by post |
| NRT 1 What's in food? | To choose foods that meet nutritional specifications. | Recap | | Part 1: 45 minutes Part 2: 60 minutes | * | Weight watchers, Student snack, Long live fruit |
| NRT 2 Changing the nutritional value of food products | That the nutritional value of products can be altered by changing the ingredients. | Extension | | 60 minutes | ** | Weight watchers, Student snack, Long live fruit |

# Resource Task Summary Tables

| Task number and title | Learning | Type of task | Links with other subjects | Time | Demand | Capability Tasks supported |
|---|---|---|---|---|---|---|
| DFPRT 1 Designing for nutrition | How to design the nutritional value of your recipes by altering the ingredients. | Extension | | 60 minutes | ** | Weight watchers, Young eaters, Frozen deliveries |
| DFPRT 2 Designing for flavour and odour | How to change the flavour and odour of foods with the ingredients that you use. | New | | 90 minutes | ** | Young eaters, Frozen deliveries |
| DFPRT 3 Designing for colour | How to control the colour of foods and investigate the effect of colour on consumer preference. | New | Science | 60 minutes | * | Young eaters, Frozen deliveries |
| DFPRT 4 Designing for texture | How to control the texture of foods by varying quantities of ingredients, cooking methods and adding extra ingredients. | New | | 90 minutes | ** | Student snack, Young eaters |
| DFPRT 5 Designing for finish | How to control the finish on a food product by altering the surface presentation. | New | | 45 minutes plus 120 minutes proving time | * | Frozen deliveries, Luxury cakes, Confectionery by post |
| DFPRT 6 Designing for shelf life | How products can be kept for a longer time by treating them in a special way. | New | | 40 minutes | ** | Can be useful to support a variety of tasks |
| DFPRT 7 Designing for cost | How to control the cost of a recipe by changing the ingredients or type of ingredients used. | New | Maths, IT | 40 minutes | *** | Soup kitchen |
| FPRT 1 Batch production and systems thinking | To plan and carry out a batch production system that is safe and quality assured. | New | | 120 minutes | *** | Air travel special diets, Soup kitchen, New breads, Better than a sandwich |
| FPRT 2 Biotechnology in the food industry | The importance of biotechnology; how to produce a prototype product using biotechnology principles. | New | Science | Part 1: 30 minutes Part 2: 120 minutes | *** | Back to your roots |
| PART 1 Comparing a collection of food products | To extend your understanding of how to investigate products. | Recap and extension | | 45 minutes | *** | Young eaters, Frozen deliveries, Long live fruit |
| FSRT 1 Breaking the chain | Some main causes of food poisoning, how you can prevent the spread of food poisoning and what food agencies are involved in monitoring food retail outlets. | New | Science | 90 minutes | * | Air travel special diets, Frozen deliveries, Luxury cakes Confectionery by post |
| FSRT 2 Labelling: who needs it? | To distinguish between the various types of information given on a label and to determine its value to the manufacturer, the retailer and the consumer. | Extension | | 60 minutes | ** | Weight watchers, Young eaters, Frozen deliveries |
| HSRT 1 Ensuring safety in an unfamiliar situation | To revise and extend your understanding of how to be safe, and ensure the safety of others. | Recap and extension | | 45 minutes | ** | Air travel special diets |

# Part 2

Capability Tasks for 14–16 year-olds

# Capability Task Summary Tables

| Line of interest | Task title | Nature of product | Useful Resource Tasks | Useful Case Studies |
|---|---|---|---|---|
| Special diets | Air travel special diets | **From the exploration:** A detailed report on two different types of special diets. A report on an airline catering factory visit or video "Food on the Move". An investigation into which foods re-heat successfully. A preliminary specification for an airline meal and a named special diet.<br>**For the production and promotion:** A selection of meal ideas which are evaluated against the preliminary specification. A detailed specification for the final product, plus a record of a system for quality control.<br>**Possible products:** A meal which includes: a starter, a main dish, one or two side dishes, a dessert, plus associated menu card and preparation instructions for cabin crew. | SRT 1 Identifying needs and likes<br>SRT 2 Questionnaires<br>SRT 3 Design briefs and specifications<br>CRT 4 Communicating production methods<br>FPRT 1 Batch production<br>FSRT 1 Food poisoning<br>HSRT 1 Ensuring safety in an unfamiliar situation<br>Note sensory analysis resource tasks SRT 6, 8 and 9 can be used if necessary<br>CRT 1 Presenting information about food products | Soup, beautiful soup |
| Special diets | Weight watchers | **From the exploration:** Information on the dietary needs of slimmers. A report on existing products, including attribute analysis, to develop ideas for the new product line. A preliminary specification of a new product. A report on the packaging used to promote slimming diet products.<br>**For the production:** A selection of product ideas which are evaluated against the product specification. A detailed specification for the final product, a nutritional analysis of the product.<br>**Possible products:** As a prototype, new products may include: chilled ready meals, biscuits or other snacks, soups, desserts, plus prototype packaging complete with visuals and user information. | SRT 1 Identifying needs and likes<br>SRT 4 Questionnaires<br>STR 5 Attribute analysis<br>PART 1 Examining a collection of products<br>NRT 1 What's in food<br>NRT 2 Changing nutritional value of food products<br>DFPRT 1 Nutrition<br>CRT 1 Presenting information about food products<br>CRT 2 Exploring packaging<br>CRT 3 Developing the stand out factor<br>FSRT 2 Looking at labels | Soup, beautiful soup<br>Making minced meat<br>Cool control |
| For the young | Young eaters | **From the exploration:** A report on food products available for children aged 1–3 years; a summary of the dietary requirements of children aged 1–3 years; a report on children's preferences; a preliminary specification for the food product.<br>**For the production and promotion:** A selection of product ideas which are evaluated against the preliminary specification; a detailed specification for the final product; a nutritional analysis of the product: sample packaging; sample full-page advertisements for good eating, magazines. | SRT 1 Identifying needs and likes<br>SRT 8 Performance specification and user trips<br>DFPRT 1 Nutrition<br>PART 1 Examining a collection of food products<br>SRT 4 Brain storming<br>DFPRT 2 Flavour and odour<br>DFPRT 3 Colour<br>DFPRT 4 Texture | Copper and you |

| Line of interest | Task title | Nature of product | Useful Resource Tasks | Useful Case Studies |
|---|---|---|---|---|
| For the young | Young eaters | **Possible products:** Main courses e.g. tomato and beef pasta, chicken bake with potato topping, vegetable savoury crumble; Desserts e.g. fresh fruit compotes, fruit milk shakes, fresh fruit slices. | FSRT 1 Food poisoning<br>CRT 1 Presenting information about food products<br>CRT 2 Exploring packaging<br>CRT 3 Developing the stand out factor<br>FSRT 2 Looking at labels | Wrap it up<br>Embedded energy |
| For the elderly | Frozen deliveries | **From the exploration:** A report on existing products aimed at this target group, perhaps as a result of a visit to Meals on Wheels; a report on a visit to a food factory to examine large scale food processing; a summary of the dietary requirements of the elderly; a report on the effects of freezing on foodstuffs; a preliminary specification for the new product.<br>**For the production and promotion:** A report on suitable production systems to supply in bulk; a detailed specification for the final product; packaging materials, storage and re-heating information; promotional material to be included in the catalogue.<br>**Possible products:** Fish and vegetable pie, pasta and vegetable medley, fruit sponge pudding. | SRT 1 Identifying needs and likes<br>SRT 8 Performance specification and user trips<br>DFPRT 1 Nutrition<br>PART 1 Examining a collection of food products<br>SRT 4 Brain storming<br>DFPRT 2 Flavour and odour<br>DFPRT 3 Colour<br>DFPRT 5 Finish<br>FSRT 1 Food poisoning<br>CRT 1 Presenting information about food products<br>CRT 2 Exploring packaging<br>CRT 3 Developing the stand out factor<br>FSRT 2 Looking at labels | Embedded energy<br>Soup, beautiful soup<br>Wrap it up |
| For those at risk | Student snack | **From the exploration:** A report on a visit to a local Student Union canteen including analysis of existing meals; a report on the constraints facing students based on an interview with Student Union officer. Consideration of the effects of storage and re-heating on possible food products; a preliminary specification for the snack product.<br>**For the production and display:** A report on suitable production systems; a report on the suitability of identified food products; a detailed specification for the final product, sample products, display material.<br>**Possible products:** Pasties, samosas, filled pitta breads, rolls, quiches. | SRT 1 Identifying needs and likes<br>SRT 2 Questionnaires<br>NRT 1 What's in food<br>NRT 2 Changing nutritional value of food products<br>CRT 1 Presenting information about products<br>FCRT 2 Sets<br>DFPRT 4 Texture | Information<br>– the power<br>to change lives |

# Capability Task Summary Tables

| Line of interest | Task title | Nature of product | Useful Resource Tasks | Useful Case Studies |
|---|---|---|---|---|
| For those at risk | Soup kitchen | **From the exploration:** A report on a talk from a local charity involved with the homeless or a summary of information from Crisis at Christmas and similar charities indicating the funds likely to be available for providing free food; a preliminary specification for the product. **For the production:** A report on a suitable production system; a detailed specification for the final product; sample products including packaging; a write up of the fund raising for a homeless publication such as Big Issue with the proceeds going to a charity. **Possible products:** Hot food from the kitchen: soups, stews, pasties, samosas, hot filled rolls, hot filled breads; food to take away: sandwiches, filled rolls, snack bars. | SRT 1 Identifying needs and likes<br>SRT 7 Evaluating Winners and losers and appropriateness<br>DFPRT 7 Cost<br>FPRT 1 Batch production<br>SRT 9 Evaluation by attribute profile<br>CRT 2 Exploring packaging | Copper and you<br>Wrap it up |
| Primary foods | Long live fruit | **From the exploration:** A report about the drying process for fruit; a report on existing products, including attribute analyses, to develop ideas for a new product line that repositions dried fruit as a concept; a preliminary specification of two new products. (1) A dried fruit snack (2) Savoury/sweet dish that has dried fruit as its basis; a report on the nutritional and other information available on dried fruit products available at present; a short case study of a recent new product – from a personal stand-point; based on supermarket visit plus other sources e.g. food magazines or radio and TV programmes. **For the production and promotion:** A selection of product ideas which are evaluated against the product specification; a detailed specification for the final product, a nutritional analysis of the product; recipe suggestions for dishes using dried fruits to be sold with the products; in store promotional display, sample packaging, and storyboard for TV commercial. **Possible products:** As a prototype new products may include originally packaged snacks: a Mango Egg! a Health Box, a Tube of Prunes, a Roll of Raisins, a Granny Leather; Chilled ready dishes: Confectionery, Side dishes, Main course meals, Fruit Soups, Desserts – all showing versatility of dried fruit. | PART 1 Examining a collection of food products<br>NRT 1 What's in food<br>NRT 2 Changing nutritional value of food products<br>CRT 1 Presenting information about food products<br>CRT 3 Developing the stand out factor | A corny story<br>Soup, beautiful soup<br>Making minced meat<br>Brand names<br>for sweeties |

| Line of interest | Task title | Nature of product | Useful Resource Tasks | Useful Case Studies |
|---|---|---|---|---|
| Primary foods | Back to your roots | **From the exploration:** A report on the range of vegetables and place of origin at present available on supermarket shelves with special attention on potatoes, parsnips, turnips, swedes and carrots – cost per portion should also be calculated; a report on British root vegetables, including methods of display and presentation, information available, current methods of cooking. Note that the chilled and frozen sections should also be examined for examples of root vegetables in use; a report on investigating the use of root vegetables for flavour, texture and appearance; a preliminary specification for a new product. **For the production and promotion:** A selection of product ideas evaluated against preliminary specification; a detailed specification for final products; a report on manufacturing possibilities for some products; presentation pack for superstore employees on British root vegetables "From English Field to Tummy – How Yummy" giving the following: display possibilities in the store, a set of cookery cards based on the products, ideas for in-store promotions eg tasting sessions. **Possible products:** Examples of root vegetable dishes such as: one to stand alone – "Just Roots"; one to serve as untraditional accompaniment e.g. Pork garnished with peppered parsnips, chilled/frozen dishes using potato that break away from the "potatoes in fixed-shapes" idea. | PART 1 Examining a collection of food products<br>SRT 1 Identifying needs and likes<br>SRT 2 Questionnaires<br>FPRT 2 Industrial production<br>SRT 6 Evaluating 1 – Ranking, preference and difference<br>CRT 1 Presenting information about food products<br>CRT 3 Developing the stand out factor | Corny story<br>Soup, beautiful soup |
| From the bakery | New breads | **From the exploration:** A report on existing products and possibilities for product development; a report on a visit to a bakery; a report on the testing and analysis of the possible ingredients and methods of processing; a preliminary specification for a new product. **For the production and promotion:** A report on suitable production systems; a report on the product development and evaluation against the product specification; a detailed specification for the final product which includes ingredients, equipment and a production schedule; sample products; promotional material. **Possible products:** New savoury or sweet bread mixtures; breads using different flours and textures; breads with different shapes and finishes. | SRT 5 Attribute analysis<br>SRT 6 Evaluation 1 – Ranking, preference and difference<br>SRT 8 Evaluation 2 – Performance specification and user trips<br>SRT 9 Evaluations 3 – Attribute profiles<br>FPRT 1 Batch production<br>CRT 1 Presenting information about food products | Bread making in Peru<br>Bread production |

# Capability Task Summary Tables

| Line of interest | Task title | Nature of product | Useful Resource Tasks | Useful Case Studies |
|---|---|---|---|---|
| From the bakery | Better than a sandwich | **From the exploration:** A report on existing products to suit a variety of cultures; a report on a visit to a bakery; a report on the testing and analysis of consumer preferences for this food range; consideration of the effects of storage and re-heating on possible food products; a preliminary specification for a new product. **For the production and promotion:** A report on suitable production systems; a report on the suitability of identified food products; a detailed specification for the final product; sample products; promotional material. **Possible products:** Filled Naan breads, pasties/samosas with various fillings, special diet pastry or bread products. | SRT 2 Questionnaires<br>SRT 4 Brainstorming<br>SRT 6 Evaluation 1 – Ranking, preference and difference<br>SRT 8 Evaluation 2 – Performance specification and user trips<br>SRT 9 Evaluations 3 – Attribute profiles<br>FPRT 1 Batch production<br>CRT 1 Presenting information about food products | Bread making in Peru<br>Bread production |
| Confectionery | Luxury cakes | **From the exploration:** A report on different sorts of party/celebration; associated confectionery and possibilities for product development; a report on a visit to a confectioners; a report on the testing and analysis of the possible ingredients and methods of processing; a preliminary specification for a new product. **For the production and marketing:** A report on the product development and evaluation against the product specification; a detailed specification for the final product; packaging and promotional material. **Possible products:** Small cakes by a variety of methods: creamed, rubbed in, whisked, melted; flavour enhanced by a variety of methods: spices, fruit, honey, shaped by a variety of methods: moulding, cutting, layering, rolling, decorated by a variety of methods: spun sugar, butter icing, sugar icing, marzipan, chocolate. | SRT 1 Identifying needs and likes<br>SRT 2 Questionnaire<br>SRT 7 Evaluation 2 Winners and losers and appropriateness<br>SRT 8 Evaluation 3 Performance specification and user trips<br>DFPRT 5 Finish<br>FSRT 1 Food poisoning<br>CRT 1 Presenting information about food products | Wrap it up |
| Confectionery | Confectionery by post | **From the exploration:** A report on different sorts of party/celebration, associated confectionery and possibilities for product development; a report on a visit to a confectioners; a report on the testing and analysis of the possible ingredients and methods of processing; a preliminary specification for a new product. **For the production and marketing:** A report on suitable production systems; a report on the product development and evaluation against the product specification; a detailed specification for the final product; packaging and promotional material. **Possible products:** Shaped and decorated sweets – fudge, toffees, chocolates, fondant, chocolate-covered preserved or dried fruits; shaped and decorated biscuits; shaped and decorated marzipan; shaped and decorated ice creams. | SRT 1 Identifying needs and likes<br>SRT 2 Questionnaire<br>SRT 7 Evaluation 2 Winners and losers and appropriateness<br>SRT 8 Evaluation 3 Performance specification and user trips<br>FCRT 3 Foams<br>FCRT 4 Emulsions<br>FSRT 1 Food poisoning<br>CRT 1 Presenting information about food products.<br>In addition students may find DFPRT 5 Finish useful. | Public transport in London; background to the transport needed for mail order and local deliveries<br>Brand names for sweeties<br>Cool control |

# Air travel special diets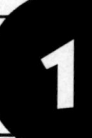

1

## A Capability Task for food technology
## Line of interest – food products for special diets

## The task

To design and make a meal that meets special dietary needs and is suitable for an airline.

## Task setting

A new airline catering company has recently been set up near Heathrow to cater for a variety of different airlines. The company requires a selection of meals that would be suitable for different special dietary needs, including vegetarians (vegans and lacto-vegetarians), coeliacs, diabetics, low-cholesterol, low-sodium diets and those required by different religions. The meals must be suitable for the requirements of airline travel, including being capable of being mass produced and reheated.

## The aims of the task

- to enable students to investigate different dietary needs
- to develop an understanding of catering
- to enable students to consider quality control and quality assurance
- to enable students to produce user information.

## Values

### technical
Students should consider the need for quality control in producing the meals, especially the importance of temperature in cooling and reheating.

### economic
Students should consider the different budgets available for meals, depending on the airline or class of travel.

### aesthetic
Students should consider the importance of the appearance and presentation of 'catered' meals.

### moral
Students should consider the reasons for respecting others' eating choices.

### social
Students should consider the influences in society that result in particular eating habits.

### environmental
Students should consider how they can minimize wastage in ready prepared 'catered' meals.

## Nature of the product

### exploration
- a detailed report on two different types of special diets
- a report on an airline catering factory visit or video 'Food on the Move'
- an investigation into which foods reheat successfully
- a preliminary specification for an airline meal and a named special diet.

### production and promotion
- a selection of meal ideas that are evaluated against the preliminary specification
- a detailed specification for the final product, including ingredients, equipment and a production schedule
- a record of a system for quality control.

### possible products
**a meal that includes:**
- a starter
- a main dish
- one or two side dishes
- a dessert

plus associated menu card and preparation instructions for the cabin crew.

## Technical knowledge and understanding

- knowledge of sensory analysis
- knowledge of the dietary requirements of people with special diets
- an understanding of a balanced meal, including nutrition, taste and texture
- an understanding of Hazard Analysis Critical Control Points.

## Specialist tools, materials and equipment

- microwave oven
- temperature probe for investigations into reheating and HACCP.

## Cross-curricular links

### maths
- accurate measurement, calculating nutritional values, ratios for portion size, calculating costs.

### science
- relevant concepts – conditions that support microbial growth.

### art
- analysis of colour to provide visually attractive meals.

### IT
- use of spreadsheets for costing and nutritional analysis
- use of DTP for reports, menu cards and instructions
- use of data logging via temperature probes.

### economic and industrial understanding
- the economics of businesses that service large industries.

## Useful Resource Tasks

**To enable students to investigate different dietary needs:**
- SRT 1 *Identifying needs and likes*
- SRT 2 *Questionnaires*
- SRT 3 *Design briefs and specifications.*

**To develop an understanding of catering:**
- CRT 4 *Communicating production methods*
- FPRT 1 *Batch production and systems thinking.*

**To enable students to consider quality control and quality assurance:**
- FSRT 1 *Breaking the chain*
- HSRT 1 *Ensuring safety in an unfamiliar situation.*
Note, sensory analysis resource tasks SRT 6, 8 and 9 can be used if necessary.

**To enable students to produce user information:**
- CRT 1 *Presenting information about food products.*

## Useful Case Studies

- Soup, beautiful soup.

## Design brief

Design and make a meal that would be suitable for an airline and meets the nutritional requirements for a specified special diet (such as vegetarian, vegans, diabetics, coeliacs, low-fat or low-cholesterol, low-sodium).

## Preliminary specification

**What the product should do:**
- provide a balanced three-course meal
- meet the requirements of a special diet
- have sufficient taste under air travel conditions.

**What the product should look like:**
- look appealing under air travel conditions.

**Other features:**
- be suitable for reheating
- be capable of withstanding movement and transportation
- be prepared, served, eaten and cleared away within the journey time
- cost an amount consistent with the airline and class of travel.

## Possible associated activities

- catering factory visit or video 'Food on the Move'
- interview manager of catering factory
- investigation of special diet requirements
- investigation of heating characteristics of frozen food using temperature probes.

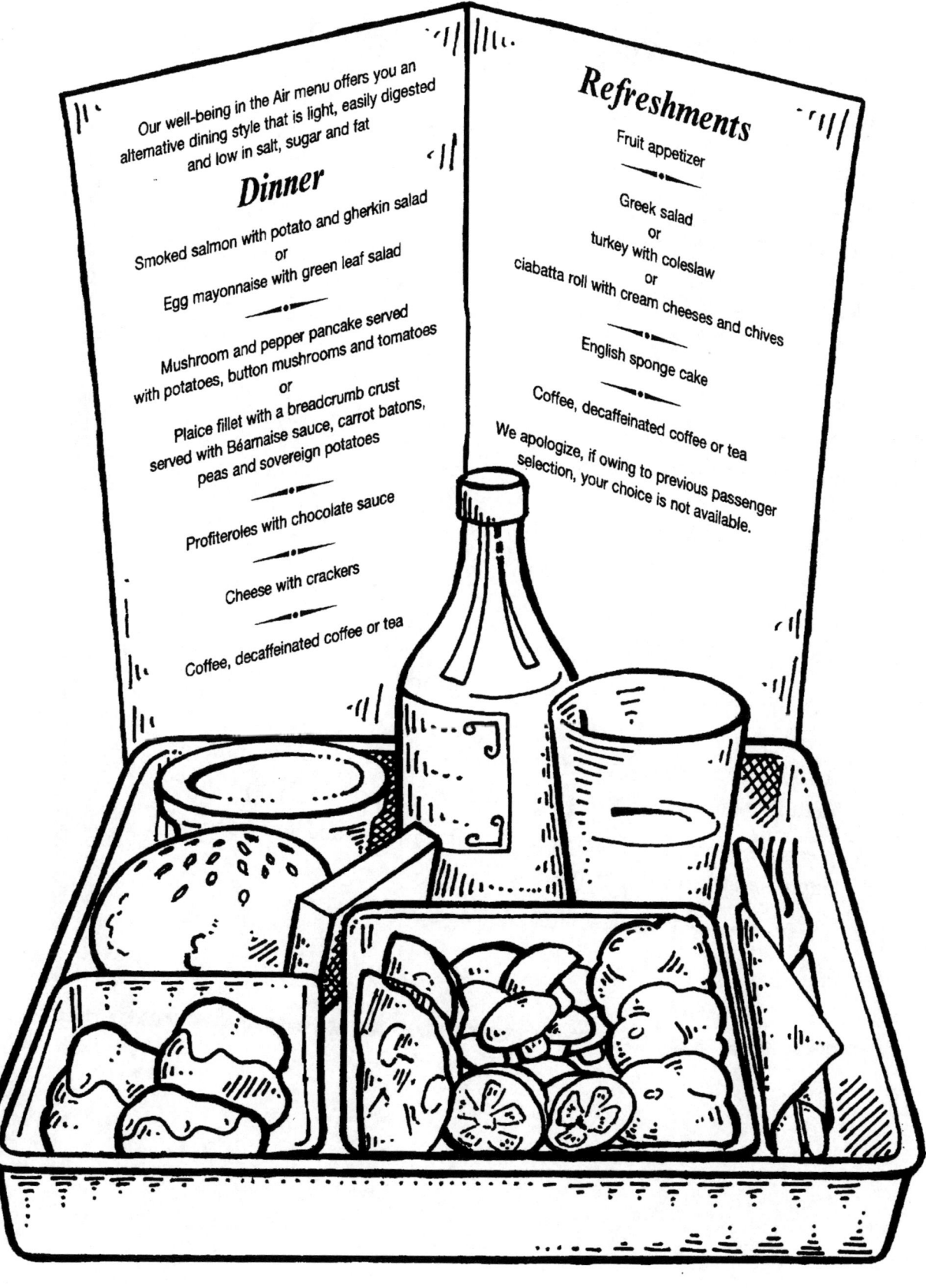

Our well-being in the Air menu offers you an alternative dining style that is light, easily digested and low in salt, sugar and fat

## Dinner

Smoked salmon with potato and gherkin salad
or
Egg mayonnaise with green leaf salad

Mushroom and pepper pancake served with potatoes, button mushrooms and tomatoes
or
Plaice fillet with a breadcrumb crust served with Béarnaise sauce, carrot batons, peas and sovereign potatoes

Profiteroles with chocolate sauce

Cheese with crackers

Coffee, decaffeinated coffee or tea

## Refreshments

Fruit appetizer

Greek salad
or
turkey with coleslaw
or
ciabatta roll with cream cheeses and chives

English sponge cake

Coffee, decaffeinated coffee or tea

We apologize, if owing to previous passenger selection, your choice is not available.

## Main dish for lacto-vegetarian:
# Mushroom and pepper pancakes

**Batter:**
100 g strong plain flour
1 large egg
300 ml milk
Approximately 5 tablespoons of oil

**Filling:**
50 g peeled and chopped mushroom
25 g butter/margarine
15 g cornflour
150 ml milk
1/2 finely chopped small red pepper
seasoning
garnish: chopped chives

**Method:**

**1** Sieve flour into mixing bowl, add egg and approximately half of the milk. Beat well. Add remaining milk.

**2** Heat butter/margarine in small saucepan. Add mushrooms and cook for 3-4 mins.

**3** Remove from heat. Blend cornflour and milk and add to mushrooms. Return to heat and stir until sauce thickens. Add chopped pepper. Cool.

**4** Heat frying pan with 1 tablespoon of oil until smoking hot. Cook approximately 6-8 thin pancakes.

**5** Fill pancakes with cooled filling. Roll and garnish.

# Weight watchers ②

## The task

To design and make to prototype stage a product suitable for people on a slimming diet.

## Task setting

A large number of people in Britain wish to lose weight. In the UK, one third of all women and half of all men are overweight and the proportions appear to be increasing. Being overweight can lead to increased risks of high blood pressure, high blood cholesterol, diabetes, coronary heart disease, respiratory diseases, gallstones and some cancers, as well as people simply feeling unhappy about their personal appearance. There are already some products on the market for people who wish to lose weight, but a major food retailer (a supermarket) wishes to develop its own range of products suitable for those who wish to lose weight.

## The aims of the task

- to enable students to understand the dietary needs of people on slimming diets and relate these to the design of a food product
- to enable students to investigate and analyse existing products on the market (such as Lean Cuisine, Boots' own products, Weight Watchers)
- to enable students to consider designing for manufacture when reviewing the feasibility of their products
- to enable students to calculate the total nutritional intake per portion of their product
- to enable students to develop appropriate packaging design and information.

## Values

### technical

Students should consider how a reduction in high-calorie ingredients (such as fats and sugars) can affect the taste and texture of finished food products.

### economic

Students should consider the growing market for slimming products and consider the costs of existing products, which will be the competition for the supermarket's range.

### aesthetic

Students should consider how the appearance of the food product on sale can influence its success in the marketplace.

### moral and social

Students should consider how our society pressurizes people to be slim, which can lead to overweight people feeling unhappy about their appearance and, in severe cases, can encourage eating disorders, such as anorexia and bulimia nervosa.

### environmental

Students should consider the role of packaging in the lifecycle of their product.

## Nature of the product

### exploration

- information on the dietary needs of slimmers
- a report on existing products, including attribute analysis, to develop ideas for the new product line
- a preliminary specification for the new product
- a report on the packaging used to promote slimming diet products.

### production

- a selection of product ideas that are evaluated against the product specification
- a detailed specification for the final product, including ingredients, equipment and a production schedule
- nutritional analysis of the product.

### possible products

**prototype new products may include:**
- chilled ready meals
- biscuits or other snacks
- soups
- desserts

plus prototype packaging, complete with visuals and user information.

## Technical knowledge and understanding

- an understanding of the nutritional requirements of slimmers
- knowledge of sensory evaluation techniques, including ranking, preference and difference tests
- knowledge of the roles of fats and sugars as ingredients in food products and how reducing these may affect the taste, texture and appearance of products
- knowledge of low-fat, reduced-calorie products that can be used as ingredients.

© The Nuffield Foundation, 1996

## Specialist tools, materials and equipment

- a range of reduced calorie products for analysis
- an ice-cream maker would be useful for frozen desserts.

## Cross-curricular links

### maths
- simple nets for packaging.

### science
- concepts – nutritional values in food materials.

### art
- composition for packaging.

### IT
- use of spreadsheets for nutritional analysis
- use of DTP for reports and packaging
- CADCAM for producing card prototype packaging.

### economic and industrial understanding
- the development of products for particular markets.

## Useful Resource Tasks

To enable students to understand the dietary needs of people on slimming diets and relate these to the design of a food product:
- SRT 1 *Identifying needs and likes*
- SRT 2 *Questionnaires.*

To enable students to investigate and analyse existing products on the market (such as Lean Cuisine, Boots' own range, Weight Watchers):
- SRT 5 *Attribute analysis*
- PART 1 *Comparing a collection of food products.*

To enable students to calculate the total nutritional intake per portion of their products:
- NRT 1 *What's in food*
- NRT 2 *Changing the nutritional value of food products*
- DFPRT 1 *Designing for nutrition.*

To enable students to develop appropriate packaging design and information:
- CRT 1 *Presenting information about food products*
- CRT 2 *Exploring packaging*
- CRT 3 *Developing that 'stand out' factor*
- FSRT 2 *Labelling: who needs it?*

## Useful Case Studies

To enable students to consider designing for manufacture when reviewing the feasibility of their products:
- Soup, beautiful soup
- Making minced meat
- Cool control.

## Design brief

Design and make a new low-calorie product that is suitable for people on slimming diets to be sold under a supermarket's own label.

## Preliminary specification

**What the product should do:**
- provide a low-calorie alternative product suitable for slimmers
- provide flavours and textures that are as appealing as the full-calorie equivalents.

**What the product should look like:**
- be as attractive, if not more attractive, than the full-calorie equivalent.

**Other features:**
- the shelf-life should be sufficiently long for it to be sold in a supermarket
- packaged as supermarket's own brand
- packaged to appeal to slimmers.

## Possible associated activities

- investigation of existing slimming products and their packaging
- comparison of reduced- and full-calorie products through sensory analysis
- investigation of recipe modification to reduce calorie content – recipes to adapt include spaghetti carbonara, lasagne, cheesecakes, apple crumble (students may find SRT 9 Evaluation by attribute profile, to be a useful starting point).

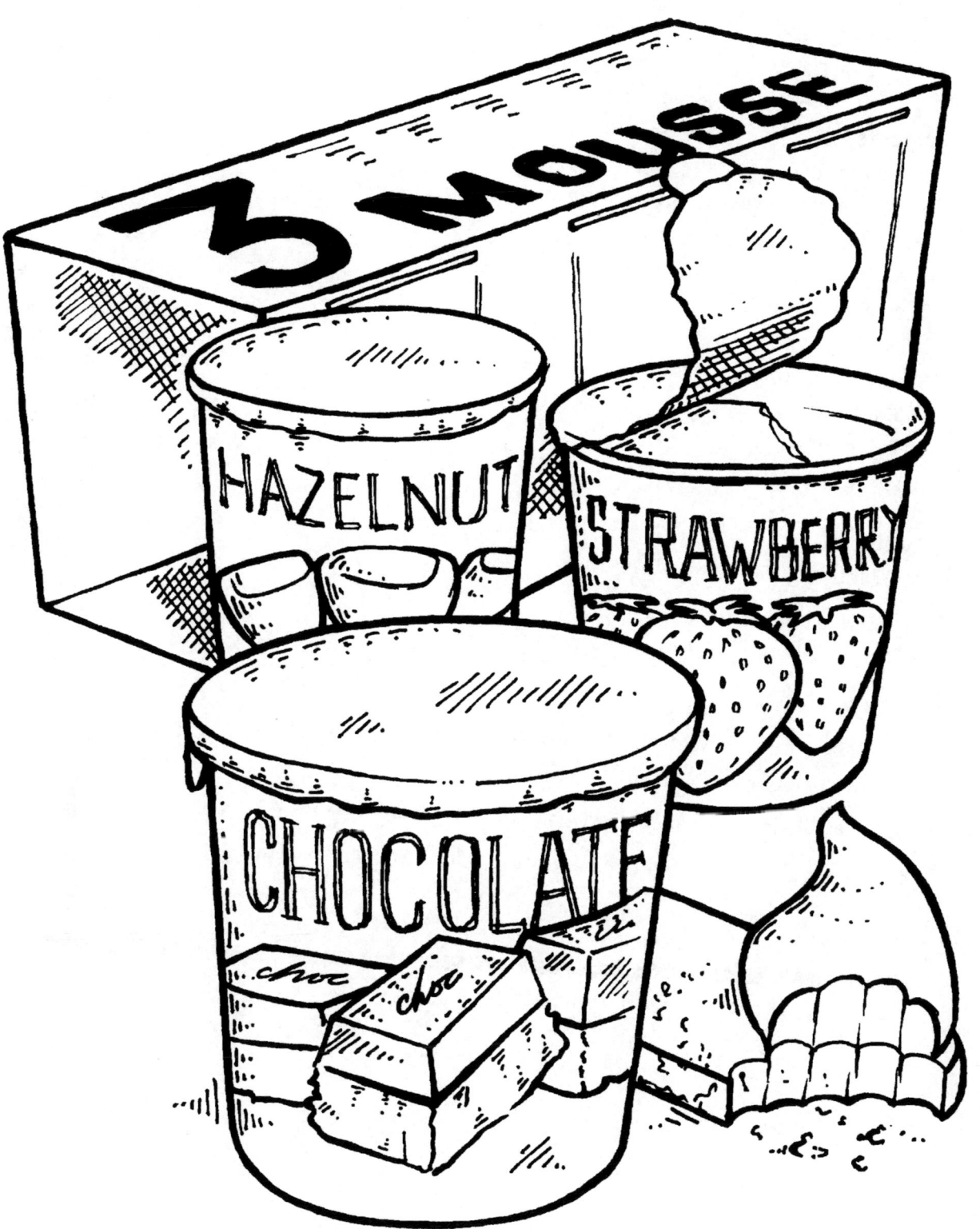

Will this style of packaging be suitable for savoury mousses?

# Salmon Mousse

**Ingredients:**

1 medium tin of salmon

1/2 pint white sauce: (1/2 pint skimmed milk, 20 g plain flour,
20 g low fat margarine, seasoning,
1/2 teaspoon dried mustard)

15 g gelatine

2-3 tablespoons water

1 tablespoon low fat mayonnaise

1 tablespoon tomato purée

50 g prawns

dash Tabasco sauce

**Method:**

**1** Lightly oil dish or mould.

**2** Break salmon into small flakes.

**3** Prepare sauce by blending method, add seasoning, purée, Tabasco and mayonnaise.

**4** Put gelatine and water in a small basin. Dissolve by standing bowl in a small saucepan of boiling water.

**5** Pour gelatine into sauce slowly, add flaked salmon and prawns.

**6** Turn into dish or mould and allow to set in a refrigerator. Turn out.

# Young eaters  (3)

## A Capability Task for food technology
## Line of interest – food products for the very young

### The task

To develop to prototype stage a food product that is suitable for the very young, to be sold in the fresh, chilled sections of a supermarket chain and that has a maximum shelf-life of three days and is suitable for home freezing.

### Task setting

With changing lifestyles, more families than ever before are dependent on ready-made meals to supplement their weekly diet. Research has shown that there is a need for a greater choice of food products designed specifically to meet the needs of very young children in the age group of one to three years.

A supermarket chain wishes to develop a range of fresh/chilled food products to provide ready-to-eat or easily prepared children's food.

### The aims of the task

- to enable students to explore the dietary/nutritional needs, alongside the food likes and dislikes, of the one to three year age group
- to enable students to investigate the current market of foods in this category in order to design improved, high-quality products
- to enable students to recognize the potential dangers of commercial ready-made food products for this age range when food hygiene and safety rules are not strictly observed

- to enable students to produce packaging and associated information, plus appropriate promotional materials that will appeal to the very young and their mothers (or the person who buys their food).

### Values

#### technical
Students should consider the need for quality assurance in food production.

#### economic
Students should consider the costs of providing both convenience and high-quality nutrition.

#### aesthetic
Students should consider how the appearance of the food product – when on sale and at the point of consumption – influences its success in the marketplace.

#### moral
Students should consider the marketing of foods that are high in potentially health-damaging foodstuffs.

#### social
Students should consider the need to encourage sensible eating practices from an early age.

#### environmental
Students should consider the use of the minimal amount of packaging materials required to protect and maintain the product.

### Nature of the product

#### exploration
- a report on food products available for children aged one to three years
- a summary of the dietary requirements of children aged one to three years
- a report on children's preferences
- a preliminary specification for the food product.

#### production and promotion
- a selection of product ideas that are evaluated against the preliminary specification
- a detailed specification for the final product, including ingredients, equipment and a production schedule

- a nutritional analysis of the product
- sample packaging
- sample full-page advertisements to appear in good food magazines.

#### possible products
- main courses, such as tomato and beef pasta, chicken bake with potato topping, savoury vegetable crumble
- desserts, such as fresh fruit compotes, fruit milk shakes and fresh fruit slices.

### Technical knowledge and understanding

- knowledge of nutritional requirements – reference to DRVs and *The Health of the Nation* document
- working knowledge of food hygiene and food safety implications (HACCP), with particular reference to chilled foods that are heated at point of consumption

- knowledge of the nutritional properties of foods
- knowledge of packaging materials.

© The Nuffield Foundation, 1996

## Specialist tools, materials and equipment

- food mixers and processors for minimal handling and mass/bulk production
- pressure cooker for sterilization

- microwave oven
- temperature probe
- packaging and suitable containers.

## Cross-curricular links

### maths

- calculation of nutritional values, ratio and proportion for portion sizes.

### science

- relevant concepts – food groups and their role in the diet.

### art

- development of the aesthetic appeal of the food products, the packaging and the advertisement.

### IT

- use of DTP for reports, summaries, packaging and advertisements
- use of spreadsheets for costing and nutritional analysis
- use of temperature probe and data handling software for safe heating investigations.

### economic and industrial understanding

- the contributions of different features to the prices of food products.

## Useful Resource Tasks

To enable students to explore the dietary/nutritional needs, alongside the food likes and dislikes, of the one to three year age group:

- SRT 1 *Identifying needs and likes*
- SRT 8 *User trip and performance specification*
- DFPRT 1 *Designing for nutrition.*

To enable students to investigate what is currently on the market in this category, in order to design improved, high-quality products

- PART 1 *Comparing a collection of food products*
- SRT 4 *Brainstorming*
- DFPRT 2 *Designing for flavour and aroma*
- DFPRT 3 *Designing for colour*
- DFPRT 4 *Designing for texture.*

To enable students to recognize the potential dangers of commercial ready-made food products for this age range when food hygiene and safety rules are not strictly observed:

- FSRT 1 *Breaking the chain.*

To enable students to produce packaging and associated information, plus appropriate promotional materials, that will appeal to the very young and their mothers (or the person who buys their food):

- CRT 1 *Presenting information about food products*
- CRT 2 *Exploring packaging*
- CRT 3 *Developing that 'stand out' factor*
- FSRT 2 *Labelling: who needs it?*

## Useful Case Studies

To enable students to explore the dietary/nutritional needs, alongside the food likes and dislikes, of the one to three year age group:

- Copper and you.

To enable students to produce packaging and associated information, plus appropriate promotional materials, that will appeal to the very young and their mothers (or the person who buys their food):

- Wrap it up
- Embedded energy.

## Design brief

To design and make a complete economical savoury food product that contains a staple food, can be served hot and is suitable for a two year old. The product will be sold from the fresh, chilled section of a leading supermarket chain and will be packaged in small individual portions with the choice of purchasing four for the price of three.

## Preliminary specification

**What the product should do:**
- provide a substantial main-meal course
- be savoury and offer an appealing mix of flavours and textures
- meet the dietary needs of children in this age group.

**What the product should look like:**
- have elements that will appeal particularly to children.

**Other features:**
- maximum shelf-life of three days
- suitable for microwave cooking
- suitable for home freezing.

It is possible to extend the specification by limiting the appeal of the product to particular groups, such as vegetarians or children with specific dietary needs, such as egg and wheat flour intolerance.

## Possible associated activities

- visit from a paediatrician
- analysis of products already on the market
- preference testing with young children
- using temperature probes to consider the use of microwave cookers for reheating food products at the point of consumption.

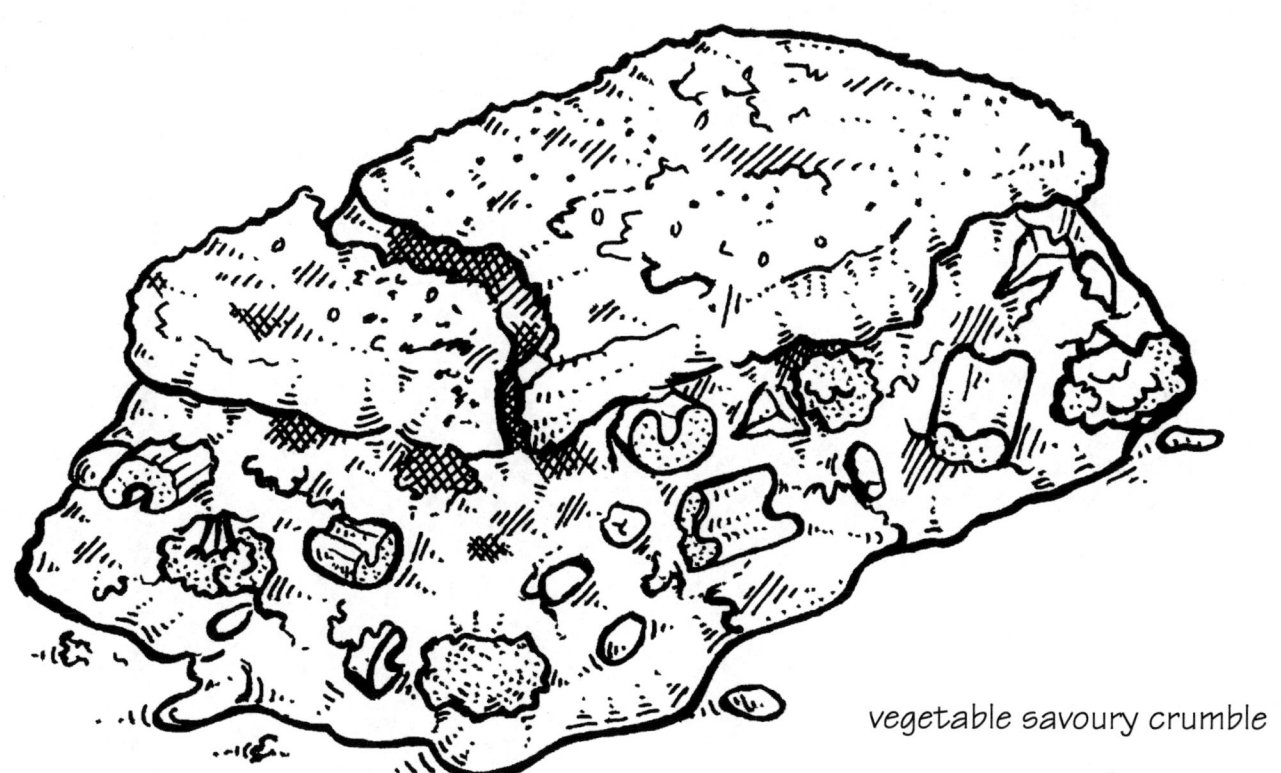

*vegetable savoury crumble*

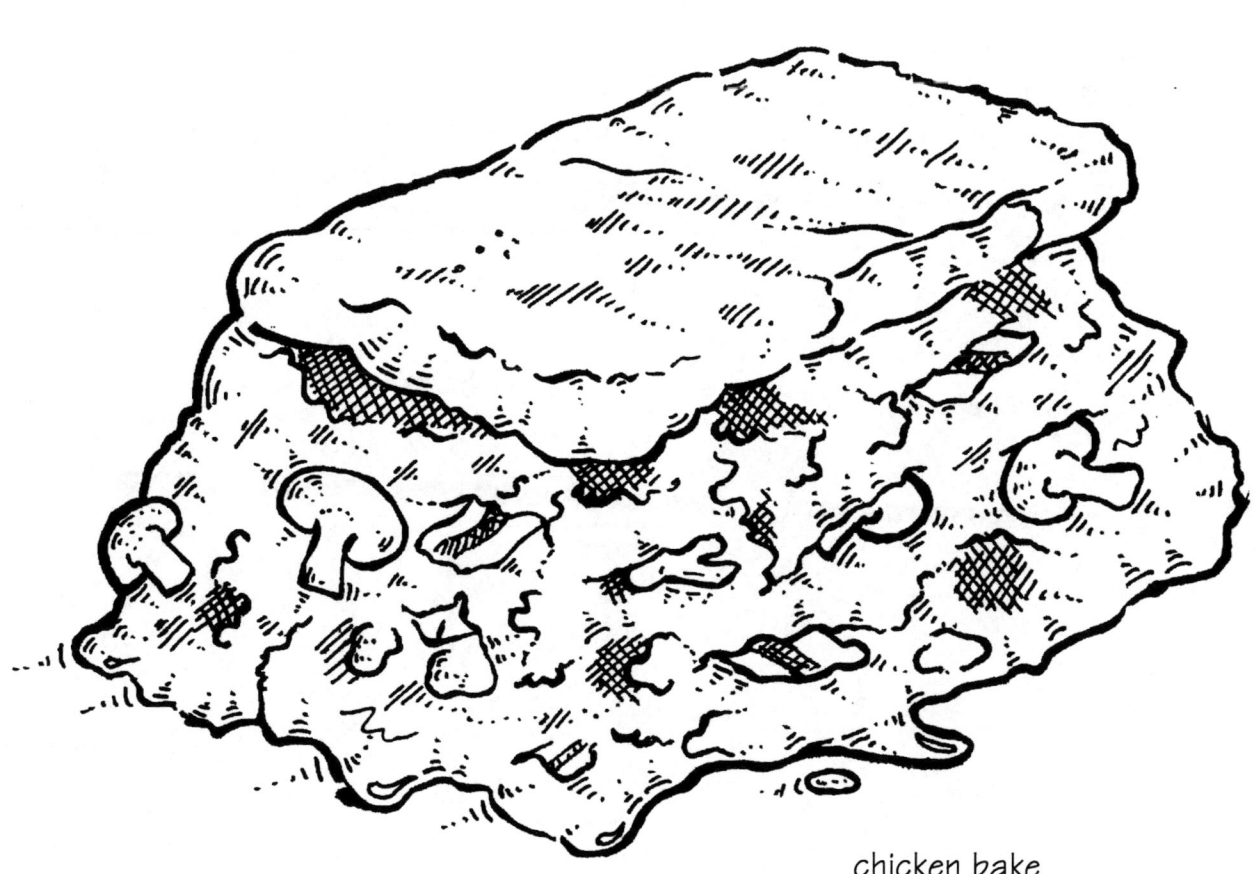

*chicken bake*

# Vegetable Savoury Crumble

**Ingredients:**

1 swede

2 carrots

2 sprigs of broccoli

1 small tin of sweetcorn

**Topping:**

10 g sesame seeds

75 g plain flour

25 g oats

50 g margarine

**Sauce:**

300 ml milk

25 g butter/margarine

25 g plain flour

25 g grated cheddar cheese

Seasoning

**Method:**

1  Oven mark 4 or 180°C.

2  Prepare sauce by roux or blending method and add the grated cheese.

3  Prepare and chop vegetables finely, add to the sauce. Pour into casserole dish.

4  Sieve flour, add oats and margarine. Rub in fat. Sprinkle over vegetable mixture. Sprinkle with sesame seeds.

5  Cook for approximately 40-50 mins until vegetables are tender.

# Frozen deliveries 4

## A Capability Task for food technology
## Line of interest – food products for the elderly

## The task

To design and make a range of frozen individual food products for the elderly to provide an alternative to the fresh meals delivered by Meals on Wheels.

## Task setting

Some recipients of Meals on Wheels would prefer to have frozen meals delivered weekly. These could be chosen at leisure from a catalogue, providing more choice in terms of meals and when they are eaten. The range of food should be economically viable, include main dishes and desserts, be suitable for freezing and provide clear instructions for the safe storage and reheating of the meal. The catalogue should promote these new food products.

## The aims of the task

- to enable students to explore the dietary/nutritional needs, alongside the food likes and dislikes, of the elderly
- to enable students to investigate the current market of foods in this category, in order to design improved high-quality products
- to enable students to consider how food products are manufactured and the effects of freezing on their quality
- to enable students to recognize the potential dangers of commercially ready-made food products for this age range when food hygiene and safety rules are not strictly observed
- to enable students to identify suitable packaging and advertising material that can be handled and understood by the elderly.

## Values

### technical
Students should consider the need for HACCP and quality control during food processing and production.

### economic
Students should consider the limited financial resources of many elderly people.

### aesthetic
Students should consider the importance of the appearance of food in tempting the elderly to eat.

### moral
Students should consider the treatment of the elderly in our society.

### social
Students should consider the role of the meal for the elderly.

### environmental
Students should consider the environmental cost of freezing.

## Nature of the product

### exploration
- a report on existing products aimed at this target group, perhaps as a result of a visit to Meals on Wheels
- a report on a visit to a food factory to examine large-scale food processing
- a summary of the dietary requirements of the elderly
- a report on the effects of freezing on foodstuffs
- a preliminary specification for the new product.

### possible products
- fish and vegetable pie
- pasta and vegetable medley
- fruit sponge pudding.

### production and promotion
- a report on suitable production systems to supply in bulk
- a detailed specification for the final product, including ingredients, equipment and a production schedule
- packaging materials, storage and reheating information
- promotional material to be included in the catalogue.

## Technical knowledge and understanding

- knowledge of the nutritional requirements of the elderly – reference to DRVs and *The Health of the Nation* document
- knowledge of the nutritional properties of food materials
- knowledge of the suitability of mass production techniques for various foods
- knowledge of the suitability of freezing for various foods
- working knowledge of food hygiene and food safety implications (HACCP) with particular reference to frozen foods that are thawed and heated at the point of consumption
- knowledge of packaging materials.

© The Nuffield Foundation, 1996

## Specialist tools, materials and equipment

- freezer
- microwave oven
- temperature probe
- packaging and suitable containers.

## Cross-curricular links

### maths
- calculation of nutritional values, ratio and proportion for portion sizes.

### science
- relevant concepts – food groups and their role in the diet.

### art
- development of the aesthetic appeal of the food products, packaging and catalogue design.

### IT
- use of DTP for reports, summaries, packaging and the catalogue
- use of spreadsheets for costing and nutritional analysis
- use of temperature probe and data handling software for safe heating investigations.

### economic and industrial understanding
- an understanding of how new markets can be identified
- the contribution of different features to the price of a food product.

## Useful Resource Tasks

To enable students to explore the dietary/nutritional needs, alongside the food likes and dislikes, of the elderly:
- SRT 1 *Identifying needs and likes*
- SRT 8 *User trip and performance specification*
- DFPRT 1 *Designing for nutrition.*

To enable students to investigate what is currently on the market in this category in order to design improved products of high quality:
- PART 1 *Comparing a collection of food products*
- SRT 4 *Brainstorming*
- DFPRT 2 *Designing for flavour and aroma*
- DFPRT 3 *Designing for colour*
- DFPRT 5 *Designing for finish.*

To enable students to recognize the potential dangers of commercial ready-made food products for this age range, when food hygiene and safety rules are not strictly observed:
- FSRT 1 Breaking the chain.

To enable students to identify suitable packaging and advertising material that can be handled and understood by the elderly:
- CRT 1 *Presenting information about food products*
- CRT 2 *Exploring packaging*
- CRT 3 *Developing that 'stand out' factor*
- FSRT 2 *Labelling: who needs it?*

## Useful Case Studies

To enable students to consider the manufacture of food products and the effects of freezing on their quality:
- Embedded energy
- Soup, beautiful soup.

To enable students to identify suitable packaging and advertising material that can be handled and understood by the elderly:
- Wrap it up.

## Design brief

To design and make a product that could be marketed, frozen and delivered to the elderly to be reheated safely and easily at their convenience. The packaging should provide clear instructions for the safe storage and reheating of the meal. The ordering catalogue should promote these new food products.

## Preliminary specification

**What the product should do:**
- conform to current dietary guidelines for the elderly
- provide an individual portion
- offer an appealing mix of flavours and textures.

**What the product should look like:**
- have elements that will appeal particularly to the elderly.

**Other features:**
- suitable for both conventional and microwave cooking
- suitable for storage in the freezer.

## Possible associated activities

- visit the Meals on Wheels service
- visit to a food factory producing 'complete dish' products
- analysis of products already on the market
- preference testing with the elderly
- investigating the freezing characteristics of different foods using temperature probes to aid consideration of the use of microwave cookers for thawing and heating food products at the point of consumption.

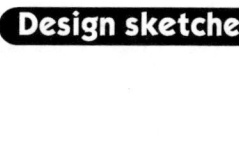

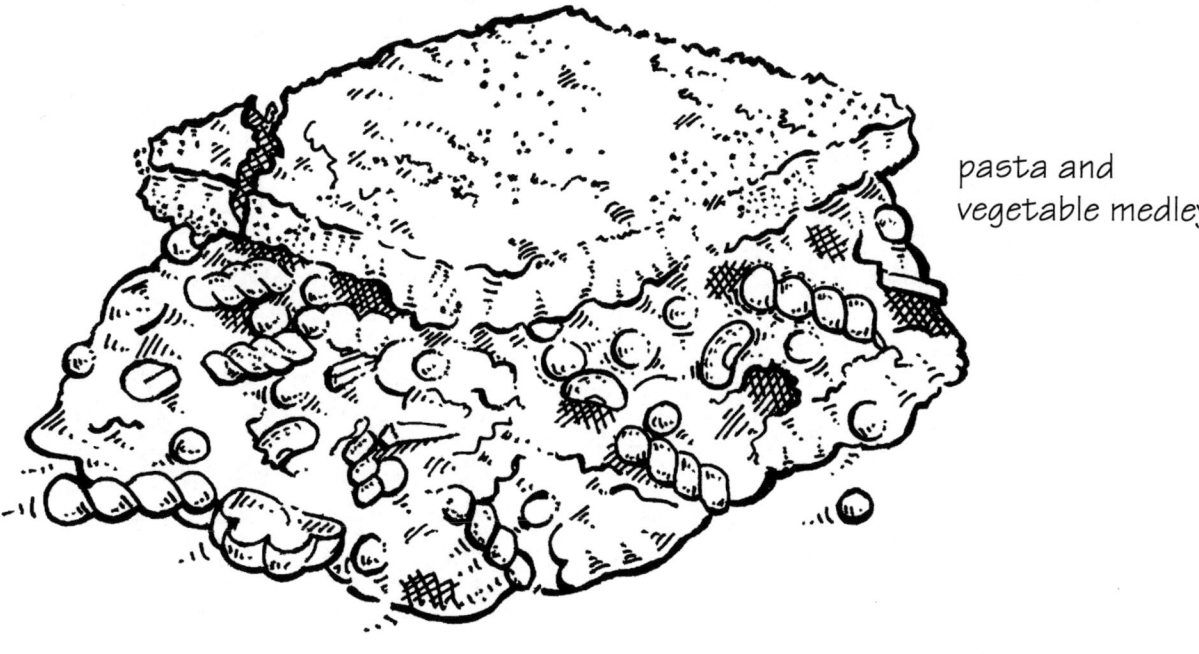

pasta and
vegetable medley

fruit sponge pudding

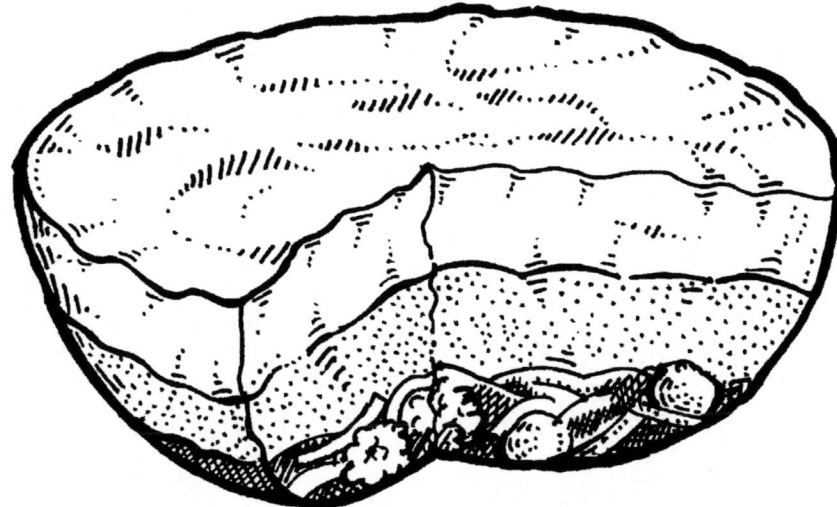

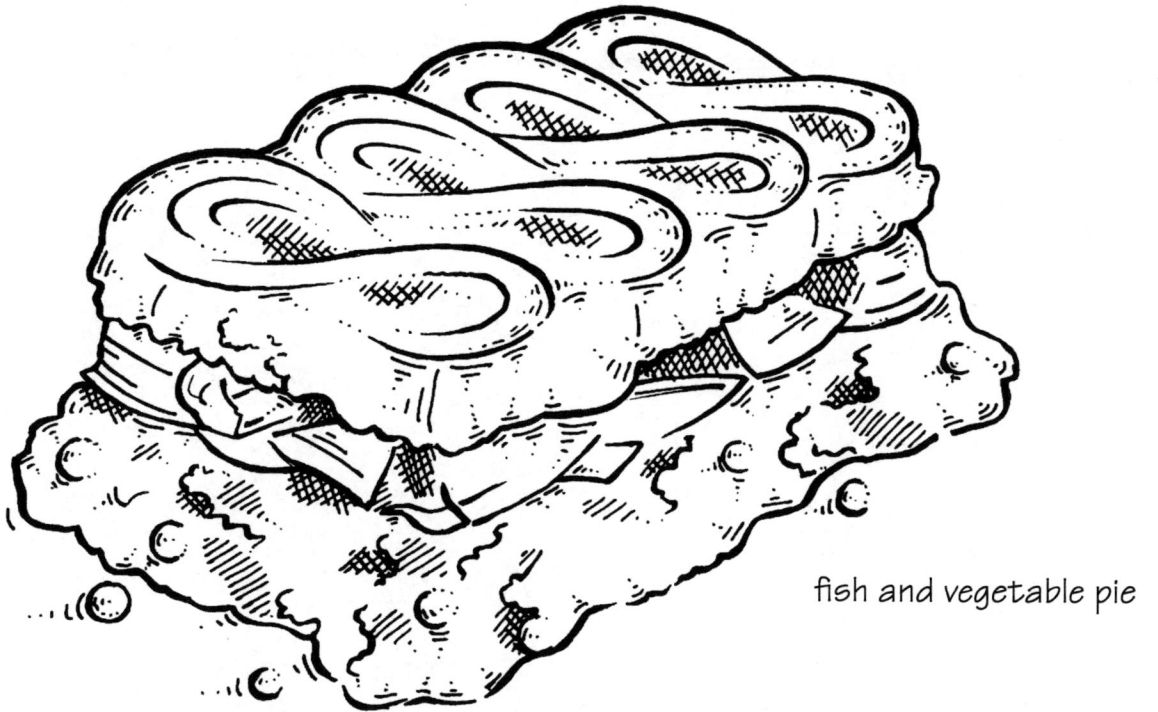

fish and vegetable pie

# Gingerbread and pear pudding

**Ingredients:**
175 g soft plain flour
2 level teaspoons ground ginger
100 g syrup
75 g soft margarine
50 g soft brown sugar
75 ml milk
1 small egg
1/2 level teaspoon bicarbonate of soda
1 small tin of halved pears

**Method:**
1  Oven mark 4 or 180°C. Grease and line a 20 cm x 25 cm tin. Arrange halved pears in base of tin.

2  Sieve flour and ginger into a mixing bowl.

3  Weigh syrup into a small saucepan, add margarine and sugar. Melt over a low heat.

4  Blend beaten egg and bicarbonate of soda into milk.

5  Pour saucepan ingredients into flour and ginger, mixing carefully. Add egg and milk. Mix well, but do not beat.

6  Pour cake batter into tin.

7  Cook for 30-40 mins. Test with a metal skewer. Turn out and cool before cutting into slices.

# Student snack  5

## The task

To develop to production stage an inexpensive, nutritious, hand-held snack food product for students, plus appropriate promotional material.

It is to be produced in a students' union canteen and purchased and consumed in a students' union bar.

## Task setting

Student grants have been cut severely and there are real economic constraints on students today, which can adversely affect their health. The student union of a local university is launching a campaign to encourage students to follow a healthy lifestyle and eat well. To support

this they wish to sell healthy, inexpensive snack foods and provide a display to be sited in the students' union building to inform students living away from home about eating healthily on a limited budget.

## The aims of the task

- to enable students to explore the difficulties encountered by those on a restricted income and the specific difficulties facing students living away from home
- to enable students to find out the dietary requirements of students aged 18 to 23 years

- to acquire and utilize display techniques
- to develop and understand the making skills required for the product.

## Values

### technical
Students should consider the means by which the product may be produced in a basic canteen.

### economic
Students should consider choosing ingredients and cooking methods that offer value for money.

### aesthetic
Students should consider the importance of appearance in a food product, even if it is inexpensive.

### moral
Students should consider the role of the students' union in promoting the health and welfare of the students.

### social
Students should consider the value of eating meals together in a student community.

### environmental
Students should consider the means by which the chosen ingredients are produced and their environmental impact.

## Nature of the product

### exploration
- a report on a visit to a local students' union canteen, including an analysis of existing meals
- a report on the constraints facing students based on an interview with a students' union officer
- consideration of the effects of storage and reheating on possible food products
- a preliminary specification for the snack product.

### production and display
- a report on suitable production systems
- a report on the suitability of the identified food products
- a detailed specification for the final product, including ingredients, equipment and a production schedule.
- sample products
- display material

### possible products
- pasties
- samosas
- filled pitta breads
- filled rolls
- quiches.

## Technical knowledge and understanding

- knowledge of sensory analysis
- knowledge of the dietary requirements of students
- knowledge of the properties of the chosen ingredients

- working knowledge of food hygiene and food safety implications
- knowledge of the suitability of batch production systems
- knowledge of graphics, of presentation techniques for display.

© The Nuffield Foundation, 1996

## Specialist tools, materials and equipment

- food processors
- microwave ovens
- temperature probes.

## Cross-curricular links

### maths

- budgeting within a student grant
- costing products and portions to include a profit margin.

### science

- relevant concepts – conditions that support microbial growth.

### art

- analysis of shape, colour and form to provide visually attractive products
- analysis of poster design for display material.

### IT

- use of spreadsheets for costing and nutritional analysis
- use of DTP to produce reports and display material
- use of data logging via temperature probes.

### economic and industrial understanding

- use of budgeting to operate within financial restraints.

## Useful Resource Tasks

To enable students to explore the difficulties encountered by those on a restricted income and the specific difficulties facing students living away from home:

- SRT 1 *Identifying needs and likes*
- SRT 2 *Questionnaires.*

To enable students to find out the dietary requirements of students aged 18 to 23 years:

- NRT 1 *What's in food*
- NRT 2 *Changing the nutritional value of food products.*

To acquire and utilize display techniques:

- CRT 1 *Presenting information about food products.*

To develop and understand the making skills required for the product:

- FCRT 2 *Making things set*
- DFPRT 4 *Designing for texture.*

## Useful Case Studies

- Information – the power to change lives.

## Design brief

To design and make an inexpensive, nutritious, hand-held snack food product for students, plus appropriate promotional material. It is to be produced in the students' union canteen and purchased and consumed in the students' union bar.

## Preliminary specification

**What the product should do:**

- provide a substantial snack meal
- offer an appealing mix of flavours and textures
- meet the dietary needs of students.

**What the product should look like:**

- be in the form of finger food.

**Other features:**

- offer value for money
- be prepared in a small canteen.

**It is possible to extend the specification by limiting the appeal of the product to particular groups:**

- lacto-vegetarian
- vegan
- specific dietary need.

## Possible associated activities

- visit to a local students' union canteen
- visit by a students' union officer
- investigation into the heating of snack products through the use of temperature probes.

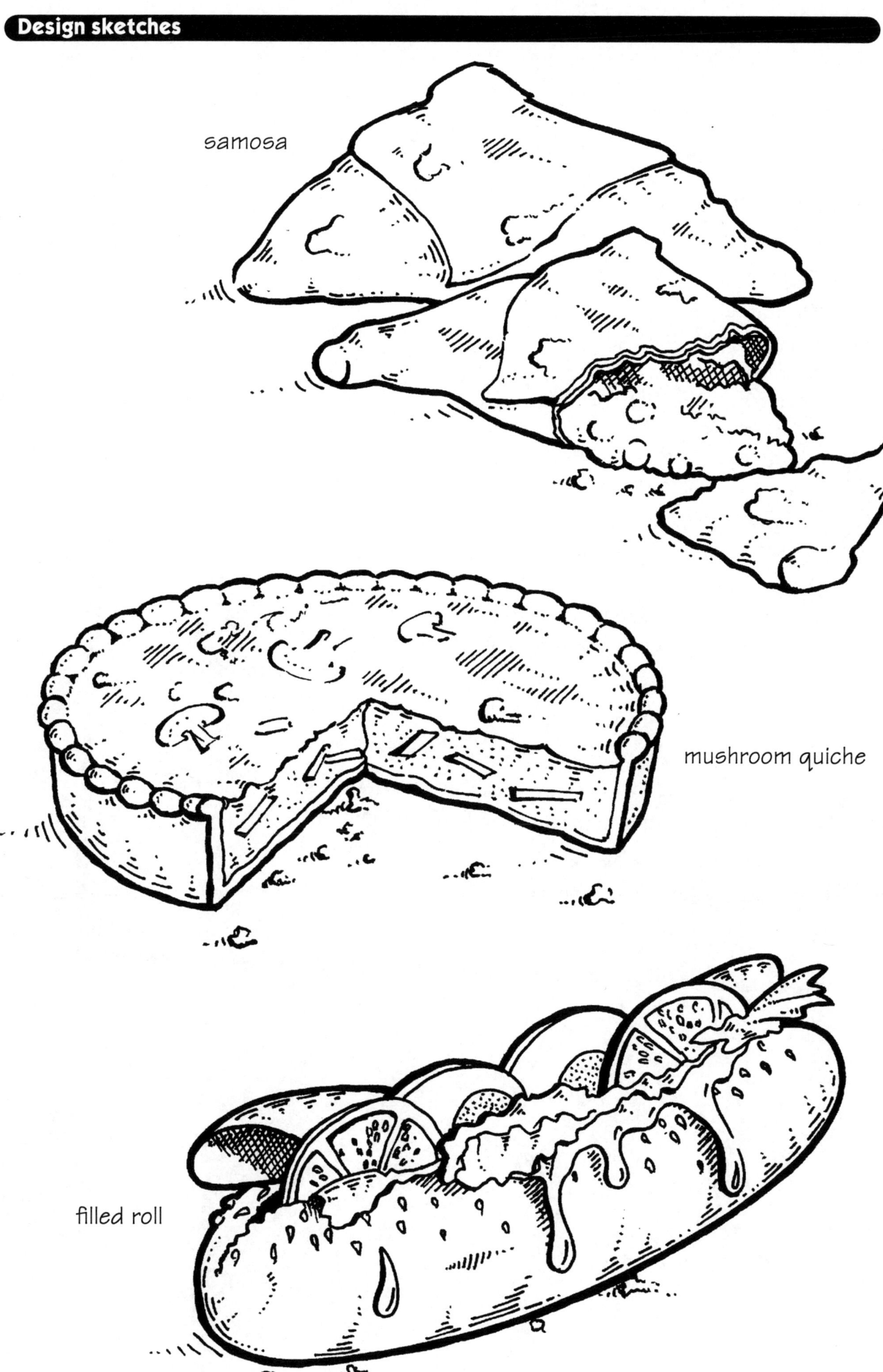

samosa

mushroom quiche

filled roll

# Pitta Packet

**Ingredients:**
6 wholemeal pittas

**Filling:**
250 g minced meat
1 small chopped onion
1 tablespoon oil
1 seeded and chopped red pepper
50 g mushrooms
1 small can of chopped tomatoes
1 teaspoon Tabasco sauce
75 g wholemeal spaghetti rings
1 teaspoon of chopped parsley

**Method**

1 Gently fry onion and mince with the oil in a pan. Add pepper, mushrooms, can of tomatoes, Tabasco sauce and seasoning. Simmer for 10 minutes.

2 Cook the pasta in a pan of fast boiling water for about 10 minutes until tender but not soft. Drain well and add to mince mixture, cool.

3 Slice pittas open and fill with the cool filling.

4 Reheat each pitta packet individually in a microwave. Each should reach a temperature of 72°C and retain this for 2 minutes. Test with a food temperature probe.

5 Sprinkle with chopped parsley.

# Soup kitchen (6)

## The task

To develop to production stage a nutritious food product suitable for serving to the homeless in a soup kitchen.

## Task setting

Homelessness is a serious problem in Great Britain today.
A local charity for the homeless has decided to set up a soup kitchen in a church hall to provide hot, nutritious food between the hours of 12.00 and 19.00 for 30 or more adults. The charity also wishes to provide a food item that can be taken away and eaten the following morning. There is the possibility that one batch of these foods could be sold at a fundraising event for the charity.

## The aims of the task

- to enable students to explore the difficulties experienced by the homeless (economic, social, physical, nutritional)
- to enable students to find out the dietary requirements of men and women of varying ages and to design appropriate meals to help meet these needs
- to work to a limited budget to produce the food products
- to enable students to design a batch production system suitable for cooking the food product for 30 or more individuals
- to develop and improve making skills for the food products
- to teach students about simple packaging.

## Values

### technical
Students should consider the ingredients required for a product high in all nutrients.

### economic
Students should consider choosing ingredients and cooking methods that offer good value for money.

### aesthetic
Students should consider the importance of appearance, aroma and flavour in making appetizing products.

### moral
Students should consider the obligations we have to help those in difficult circumstances.

### social
Students should consider the role of statutory and voluntary bodies in caring for the homeless.

### environmental
Students should consider the choice of ingredients and the impact these have on the environment (for example, new or novel sources of protein) and develop suitable packaging for the takeaway food item.

## Nature of the product

### exploration
- a report on a talk from a local charity involved with the homeless, such as the Salvation Army, or a summary of information from Crisis at Christmas and similar charities, indicating the funds likely to be available for providing free food
- a preliminary specification for the product.

### production
- a report on a suitable production system
- a detailed specification for the final product, including ingredients, equipment and a production schedule
- sample products, including packaging
- a write-up of the fundraising for a homeless publication, such as *The Big Issue,* with the proceeds going to a charity for the homeless.

### possible products
**hot food from the kitchen:**
- soups
- stews
- pasties
- samosas
- hot filled rolls
- hot filled breads.

**Food to take away:**
- sandwiches
- filled rolls
- snack bars.

## Technical knowledge and understanding

- knowledge of batch cooking and portion control
- knowledge of the dietary requirements of adults
- knowledge of the food properties of appropriate ingredients
- working knowledge of food hygiene and food safety implications (HACCP)
- knowledge of batch production systems.

© The Nuffield Foundation, 1996

## Specialist tools, materials and equipment

- microwave oven
- pressure cookers
- large-scale food processor
- temperature probe.

## Cross-curricular links

### maths
- budgeting for production costs to fit the amount of money allotted
- portion control to ensure that the food is evenly distributed
- simple nets for packaging.

### science
- relevant concepts – conditions that support microbial growth.

### art
- analysis of poster design for display materials.

### IT
- use of DTP for producing instructions for voluntary helpers who prepare the food
- use of spreadsheets for costings
- use of data logging via temperature probe.

### economic and industrial understanding
- awareness of the financial constraints encountered by local and national charities
- budgeting and profit margins.

## Useful Resource Tasks

To enable students to explore the difficulties experienced by the homeless (economic, social, physical and nutritional):
- SRT 1 *Identifying needs and likes*
- SRT 7 *Winners and losers and appropriateness.*

To enable students to work to a limited budget to produce the food products:
- DFPRT 7 *Designing for cost.*

To enable students to design a batch production system suitable for cooking the food product for 30 or more individuals:
- FPRT 1 *Batch production and systems thinking.*

To develop and improve the making skills for the food products:
- SRT 9 *Evaluation by attribute profile.*

To teach students about simple packaging:
- CRT 2 *Exploring packaging.*

## Useful Case Studies

To enable students to find out the dietary requirements of men and women of varying ages and to design appropriate meals to help meet these needs:
- Copper and you.

To teach students about simple packaging:
- Wrap it up.

## Design brief

To design and make a nutritious food product suitable for the homeless in a soup kitchen and to design and make a takeaway food product (plus packaging) to be eaten the following day.

## Preliminary specification

**What the product should do:**
- meet the dietary needs of homeless adults
- offer an appealing mix of flavours and textures.

**What the product should look like:**
- be presented in an appealing manner.

**Other features:**
- be inexpensive to produce
- be capable of being prepared in a small church hall-type kitchen.

It may be possible to extend the specification by detailing the percentage of DRV for particular nutrients that the food provides.

## Possible associated activities

- visit from a Salvation Army worker
- analysis of *The Big Issue* articles
- investigation into the safe heating of food products through use of temperature probe.

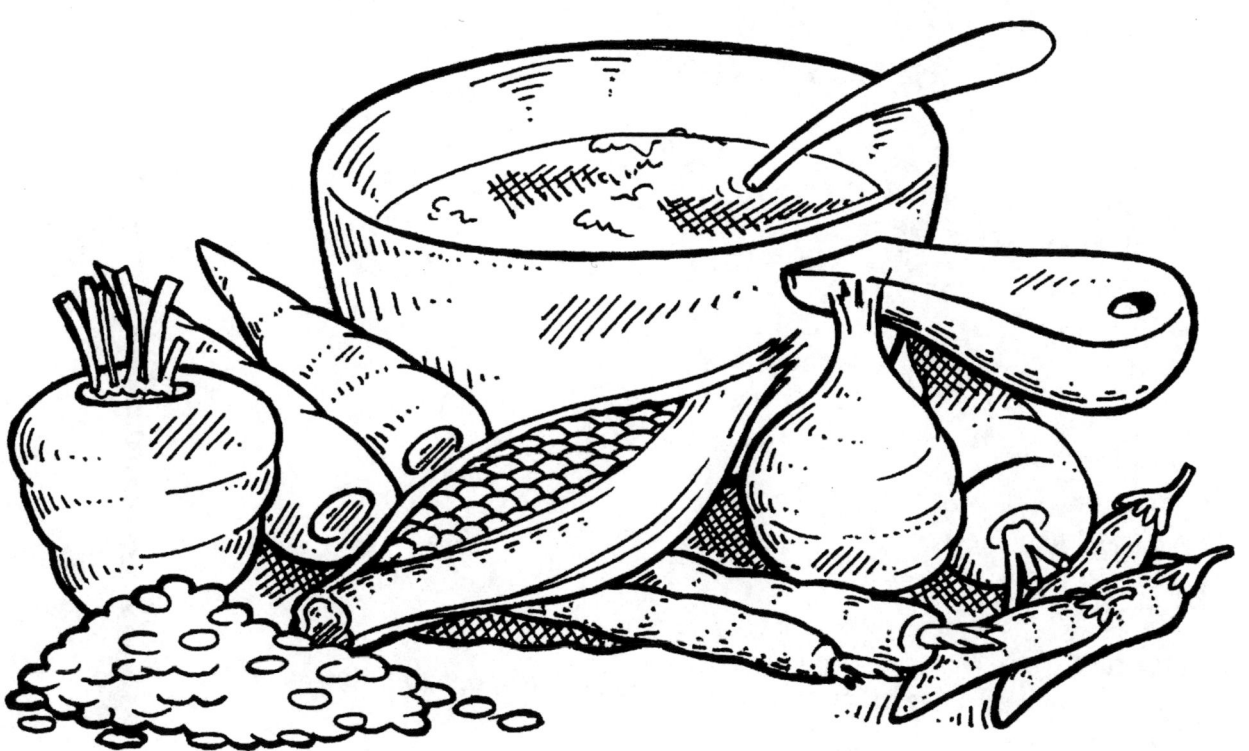

vegetable soup

# Harvest Vegetable Soup

**Ingredients:**
1 small onion
2 tablespoons oil
250 g carrot
1 medium potato
1 small green pepper, seeded and chopped
25 g lentils
25 g cornflour
200 ml milk
50 g cheddar cheese
bay leaf and seasoning

**Method:**

1  Lightly fry the peeled and chopped onion, carrots, potato in the oil until soft.

2  Add 300 ml water, lentils, seasoning and bay leaf and simmer for 30 mins.

3  Blend the cornflour with the milk and gradually add to the soup mix. Stir well until it thickens. Simmer for 5 mins then add grated cheese.

4  Serve with fresh wholemeal bread rolls.

# Long live fruit ⑦

## A Capability Task for food technology
## Line of interest – food products from primary foods

## The task

To design and make to prototype stage a product that repositions dried fruit in the marketplace.

## Task setting

The drying of fruit as a means of preservation has existed for centuries. We are all familiar with currants, raisins and cherries in a variety of food products, but all fruit is capable of being 'dried'. Apples, mangoes, bananas and prunes are all dried for sale. They are a particularly good source of fibre and are a non-fat, no added sugar food.

Dry Snax Limited is a major producer of dried fruit and is anxious to promote its products in a new, dynamic way. It would like the 'nibbling habits of the nation' to include dried fruit.

In cooking, these foods need no extra sugar, so Dry Snax would like a television and magazine promotion that emphasizes this, too.

## The aims of the task

- to enable students to understand the preservation of food, that is, fruit
- to enable students to investigate and analyse existing dried fruit products and how they are promoted
- to enable students to consider designing and making for manufacture when reviewing the feasibility of their product

- to enable students to calculate the total nutritional intake and advantages of their product
- to enable students to gain insight into the positioning and repositioning of products in the marketplace
- to enable students to develop appropriate ideas for promotion.

## Values

### technical
Students should consider the different processes involved in the preservation of foods, comparing their advantages and disadvantages.

### economic
Students should consider 'fair trade' implications for the growers/producers of the fruit – what proportion of the final profit do they receive?

### aesthetic
Students should consider how the appearance of a food product influences its sale.

### moral
Students should consider whether or not a food producer can justify deliberately stimulating demand for a new product (students should also consider the advertising standards guidelines for the promotion of new products).

### social
Students should consider the growing market for 'healthy' foods and how this is affecting what people eat.

### environmental
Students should consider the use of organic and non-organic methods of producing fruit.

## Nature of the product

### exploration
- a report on the drying process for fruit
- a report on existing products, including attribute analyses, to develop ideas for a new product line that repositions dried fruit as a concept
- a preliminary specification of two new products:
- a dried fruit snack
- savoury/sweet dish based on dried fruit
- a report on the nutritional and other information available on existing dried fruit products
- a short case study of a recent new product – from a personal standpoint – based on a supermarket visit, plus other sources, such as food magazines or radio and TV programmes.

### production and promotion
- a selection of product ideas that are evaluated against the product specification
- a detailed specification for the final product, including ingredients, equipment, the cost involved, a production schedule and a nutritional analysis of the product
- recipe suggestions for dishes using dried fruits that are to be sold with the products
- in-store promotional display, sample packaging and the storyboard for a TV commercial

### possible products
**as a prototype new products may include:**
- originally packaged snacks
  a mango egg
  a health box
  a tube of prunes
  a roll of raisins
  a granny leather
- chilled ready dishes
  confectionery
  side dishes
  main-course meals
  fruit soups
  desserts
all showing the versatility of dried fruit.

© The Nuffield Foundation, 1996

## Technical knowledge and understanding

- knowledge and understanding of how fruit is dried and its effect on taste, texture, appearance, shelf-life and nutritional values
- knowledge and understanding of the nutritional properties of dried fruit – non-fat, low sugar, high fibre – and how they meet modern nutritional requirements.

## Specialist tools, materials and equipment

- range of existing dried fruit and dried fruit products for analysis
- recent publications that contain references to the use of dried fruit
- video of commercial food promotion that looks particularly at repositioning a familiar product, such as Tango, Lucozade, OXO, Marmite
- a drying oven would be useful for student investigations.

## Cross-curricular links

### maths
- measuring changes in mass and volume caused by the drying process.

### science
- relevant concepts – conditions that support microbial growth.

### art
- what images promote dried fruit best – for example, a prune or a plum.

### IT
- use of spreadsheets for costing and nutritional analysis
- use of DTP for reports and promotional materials.

### economic and industrial understanding
- repositioning of food products in the marketplace.

## Useful Resource Tasks

To enable students to investigate and analyse existing dried fruit products and their promotion:
- PART 1 *Comparing a collection of food products.*

To enable students to calculate the total nutritional intake and advantages of their product:
- NRT 1 *What's in food*
- NRT 2 *Changing the nutritional value of food products.*

To enable students to develop appropriate ideas for promotion:
- CRT 1 *Presenting information about food products*
- CRT 3 *Developing that 'stand out' factor.*

## Useful Case Studies

To enable students to consider designing and making for manufacture when reviewing the feasibility of their product:
- A corny story
- Soup, beautiful soup
- Making minced meat.

To enable students to gain insight into the positioning and repositioning of products in the marketplace:
- Brand names for sweeties.

## Design brief

To design and make a new dried fruit product that is suitable as a low-fat, high-fibre snack and can be incorporated into a cooked dish.

## Preliminary specification

**What the product should do:**
- be based on dried fruit
- provide an alternative to current snacks.

**What the product should look like:**
- it should look fun and be compact, unusual and eye-catching.

**Other features:**
- provide a focal point for the promotion of a wider range of dried fruit products and possibilities
- inject life into a product seen mainly as a supplementary ingredient.

## Possible associated activities

- visit to a supermarket to research the place dried fruits occupy in food selling
- research into the origins of dried fruits
- research into the methods of drying
- investigation into drying of fresh fruits.

**Design sketches**

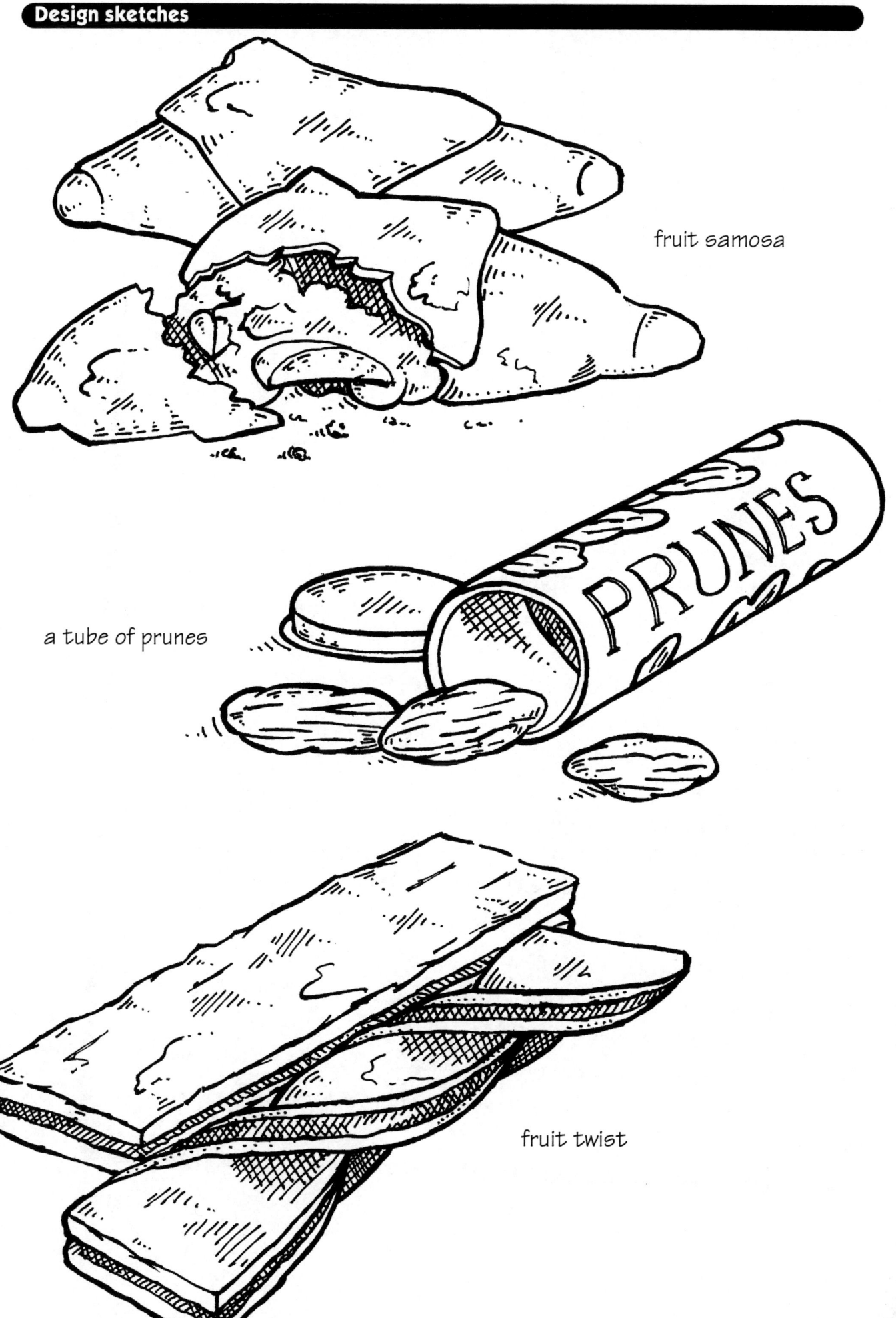

fruit samosa

a tube of prunes

PRUNES

fruit twist

# Date and Apricot Twists

**Rough Puff Pastry:**
225 g strong plain flour
pinch salt
175 g hard margarine or butter
1 teaspoon lemon juice
150 ml cold water

**Filling:**
75 g stoned and chopped dates
25 g chopped dried apricots
1/4 teaspoon cinnamon
10 g sultanas
25 g icing sugar

**Method:**

1 Prepare pastry. Sieve flour and salt into a mixing bowl.

2 Rub 25 g of the fat into the flour. Mix to a pliable dough with water and lemon juice. Knead and cool for 10-15 mins.

3 Place remaining fat between 2 pieces of greaseproof paper and beat to a flat cake with a rolling pin. Cool.

4 Roll out dough to a rectangle, place the fat in the middle. Fold up like a parcel and turn over.

5 Roll out dough into an oblong, fold into 3 and make a half turn to bring the open end towards you.

6 Repeat this 3 times to make 3 turns of the pastry.

7 Chill for at least 10 mins before use.

8 Combine ingredients for filling.

9 Roll pastry out into an oblong. Divide into 2 and spread filling on one half. Cover with remaining pastry.

10 Cut into strips and twist each strip before putting on to a cool baking tray.

11 Bake in oven mark 8 or 220°C for 7-10 mins. Dredge with icing sugar.

# Back to your roots

## A Capability Task for food technology
## Line of interest – food products from primary foods

## The task

To design and make to prototype stage a range of products that repositions British root vegetables in the marketplace.

## Task setting

Supermarkets offer a wide range of vegetables, from the exotic to the ordinary. Many of these vegetables are imported, yet we grow many vegetables ourselves. Particularly during the winter months, if we could use our own home-grown root vegetables, we could have economical, nutritional and delicious meals at a fraction of the cost of using expensive imported vegetables. Why are some vegetables fashionable and therefore in demand?

A major supermarket chain wishes to develop a range of cookery cards that promote British root vegetables. As part of the promotion, there will be sampling sessions at all its branches. The company wants the emphasis to be on the nutritional, low-fat, high-volume potential of the products – 'Filling, not fattening' is the slogan. The company is well aware that the image of root vegetables is not an exciting one at the moment.

## The aims of the task

- to enable students to investigate and analyse existing products (ranges of vegetables) and their promotion (such as that given to products by Sainsbury or Tesco)

- to enable students to consider designing for manufacture when reviewing the feasibility of their products
- to enable students to develop appropriate testing techniques
- to enable students to develop promotion for a product range.

## Values

### technical
Students should consider which food materials produce high-volume, lower-calorie products and how such materials may be made to look attractive.

### economic
Students should consider the cost of using home-grown root vegetables as a staple in the diet compared to imported vegetables, as a weekly/monthly/yearly cost.

### aesthetic
Students should consider the transformation from soil-covered root to edible delicacy in developing the promotional material.

### moral
Students should consider whether or not a supermarket chain can justify deliberately stimulating demand for a particular product.

### social
Students should consider the place of gardening and allotments in people's lifestyles.

### environmental
Students should consider the implications – cost, flavour, appearance – of organically grown root vegetables as opposed to commercially grown ones.

## Nature of the product

### exploration
- a report on the places of origin and range of vegetables at present available on supermarket shelves, with special attention being paid to potatoes, parsnips, turnips, swedes and carrots (the cost per portion should also be calculated)
- a report on the current state of play of British root vegetables, including methods of display and presentation, information available, current methods of cooking (note that the chilled and frozen sections should also be examined for examples of root vegetables in use)
- a report on investigating how root vegetables can be used for flavour, texture and appearance
- a preliminary specification for a new product.

### production and promotion
- a selection of product ideas that are evaluated against the product specification
- a detailed specification for final products, including ingredients, equipment and a production schedule
- a report on possible manufacturing possibilities for some products

- presentation pack for superstore employees for British root vegetables – 'From English field to tummy – how yummy' – giving the following:
- display possibilities in the store
- a set of cookery cards based on the products
- ideas for in-store promotions, such as tasting sessions.

### possible products
**examples of root vegetable dishes, such as:**
- one to stand alone – 'just roots'
- one to serve as an untraditional accompaniment, such as pork garnished with peppered parsnips
- chilled or frozen dishes using potatoes that break away from the 'potatoes in fixed shapes' idea.

© The Nuffield Foundation, 1996

## Technical knowledge and understanding

- knowledge of sensory analysis
- knowledge and understanding of the nutritional values of root vegetables and the role they play at present in our diet
- knowledge and understanding of cookery methods and processes that will explore the potential of these vegetables
- knowledge of dietary analysis of ingredients and their value to the consumer
- knowledge of manufacturing systems for root vegetables.

## Specialist tools, materials and equipment

- a range of vegetables that includes British root vegetables to examine, prepare, taste
- a selection of current writing on vegetable cooking
- menus from top restaurants to show how root vegetables are offered at present.

## Cross-curricular links

### maths

- accurate measurement, calculating nutritional values, ratios for portion sizes.

### science

- relevant concepts – the effects of cooking methods on food materials in roots.

### art

- use of images in packaging and promotion.

### IT

- use of spreadsheets for costing and nutritional analysis
- use of DTP for reports and promotional materials.

### economic and industrial understanding

- repositioning of products in the marketplace
- the role of imports and exports.

## Useful Resource Tasks

To enable students to investigate and analyse existing products (ranges of vegetables) and their promotion (such as how Sainsbury or Tesco do this):
- PART 1 *Comparing a collection of food products.*

To enable students to understand people's preferences regarding vegetable purchases and cooking:
- SRT 1 *Identifying needs and likes*
- SRT 2 *Questionnaires.*

To enable students to develop appropriate testing techniques:
- SRT 6 *Evaluating using ranking, preference and difference tests.*

To enable students to develop promotion for a product range:
- CRT 1 *Presenting information about food products*
- CRT 3 *Developing that 'stand out' factor.*

## Useful Case Studies

To enable students to consider designing for manufacture when reviewing the feasibility of their products:
- A corny story
- Soup, beautiful soup.

## Design brief

Design and make two new root vegetable dishes that:
- stand alone as a complete meal for a modern family
- serve as an interesting accompaniment to a main course.

Use these as the basis for a display/promotion/sampling exercise in a supermarket and for inclusion in a set of promotional cookery cards.

## Preliminary specification

**What the product should do:**
- compare favourably with more exotic imported products.
- be based on root vegetables
- provide an accompaniment to a main course
- provide a stand alone main meal
- be surprising – not just a load of mash.

**What the product should look like:**
- be attractive and appealing.

**Other features:**
- broaden the appeal of root vegetables – particularly with regard to the 'filling, not fattening' idea
- inject life into a product seen mainly as an accompaniment.

## Possible associated activities

- visit to supermarket to research the placing of root vegetables
- visit a root vegetable processing plant
- brainstorm the phrase 'Beyond the dirty knobbles' – what ways are there to promote our roots?
- brainstorm product ideas:

root slices?
roots à la Grecque?
roots 'n' shoots?
root pie?
root bread?

© The Nuffield Foundation, 1996

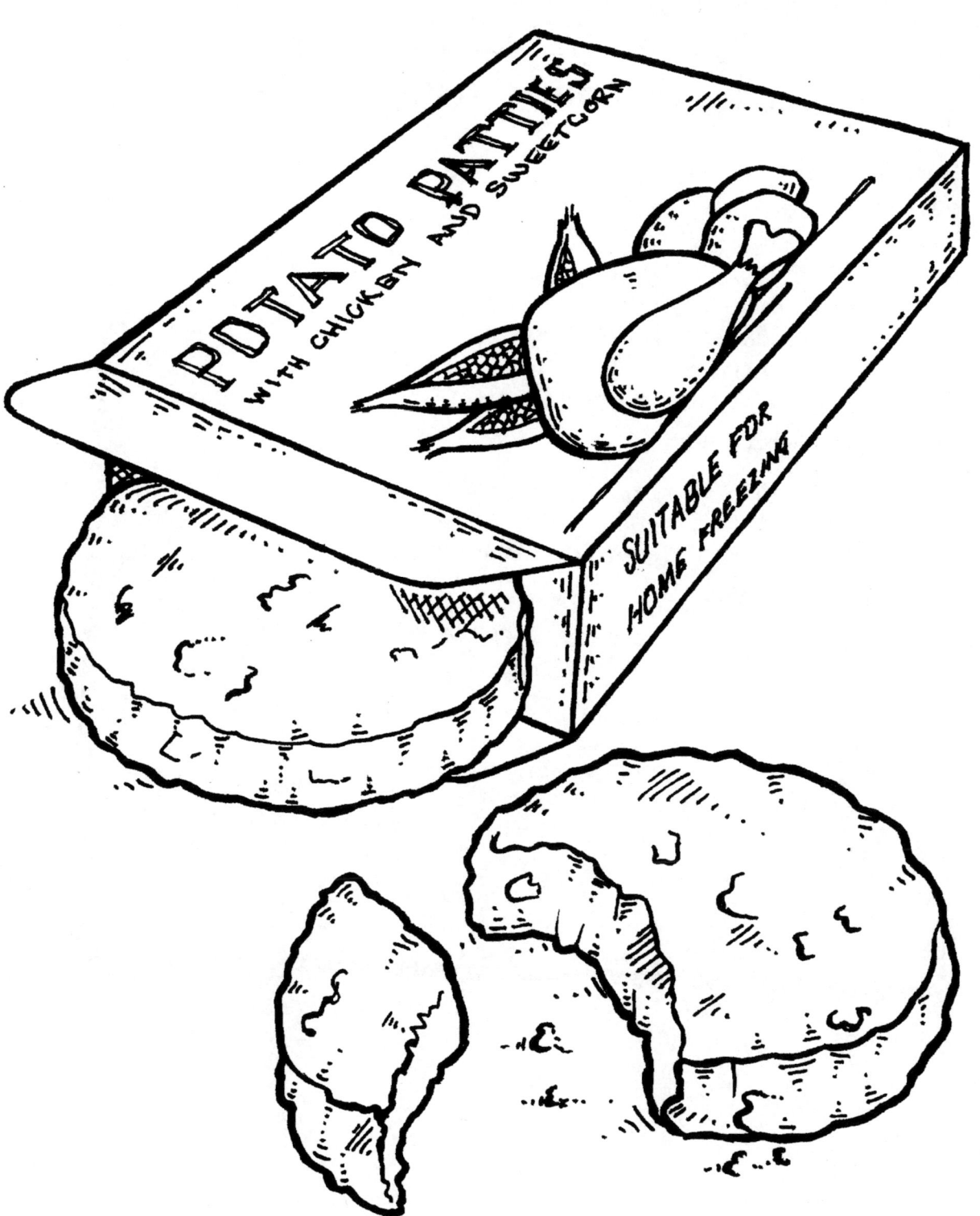

a range of potato cakes with extra ingredients

# Potato, chicken and sweetcorn cakes

**Ingredients:**
200 ml milk
2 eggs
125 g flour
pepper and salt
450 g of peeled and coarsely grated potato
1 large thinly sliced onion
225 g cooked chicken, finely chopped
1 small tin of sweetcorn
oil for frying

**Method:**

1 Whisk eggs and milk together, beat in flour and salt until smooth. Chill in refrigerator.

2 Blanch potatoes and onion in a pan of boiling water for 2-3 mins. Drain well and press out additional liquid.

3 Stir chicken into the batter with the sweetcorn, potato and onion. Add seasoning.

4 Heat 2 tablespoons of oil in a frying pan. Spoon heaped tablespoons of the mixture into a pan, flatten and fry for about 4 mins on each side. Drain on kitchen paper.

# New breads  9

## A Capability Task for food technology
## Line of interest – food products from the bakery

## The task

To design and make a range of specialized bread products and develop appropriate promotion.

## Task setting

A small family business bakery sells bread, cakes and sandwiches. To become more profitable, it has decided to bake and sell more specialized bakery products.

## The aims of the task

- to enable students to analyse products to inform their designing and making
- to develop an understanding of bread products
- to enable students to develop high-quality making skills and consider small batch production issues
- to enable students to develop promotion for a product range.

## Values

### technical
Students should consider the need for hazard analysis and quality control during food processing and production.

### economic
Students should consider the contribution of specialized products to the overall profitability of a small business.

### aesthetic
Students should consider the visual aspects of food products that might be derived from cultural influences.

### moral
Students should consider whether or not a small business can justify deliberately creating a market for a new line of products.

### social
Students should consider the role of a small bakery in the life of a local community.

### environmental
Students should consider world issues of ingredient cultivation and development together with the effects of manufacturing processes on the environment today.

## Nature of the product

### exploration
- a report on existing products and possibilities for product development
- a report on a visit to a bakery
- a report on the testing and analysis of the possible ingredients and methods of processing
- a preliminary specification for a new product.

### production and promotion
- a report on suitable production systems
- a report on the product development and that is evaluated against the product specification
- a detailed specification for the final product, including ingredients, equipment and a production schedule
- sample products
- promotional material.

### possible products
- new savoury or sweet bread mixtures
- breads made using different flours and textures
- breads with different shapes and finishes.

## Technical knowledge and understanding

- knowledge of sensory analysis
- knowledge of principles and methods used for making bread
- knowledge of the properties of ingredients, the methods that should be used to incorporate them and their effects on basic bread mixtures
- knowledge of dietary analysis of ingredients and their value to the consumer
- knowledge of the suitability of batch production systems.

© The Nuffield Foundation, 1996

## Specialist tools, materials and equipment

- a wide range of flours
- food processors with dough-kneading accessories.

## Cross-curricular links

### maths
- accurate measurement, calculating nutritional values, ratios for portion size.

### science
- relevant concepts – raising agents as chemical reactions that generate gases.

### art
- analysis of form to provide shape of bread products.

### IT
- use of spreadsheets for costing and nutritional analysis
- use of DTP for reports and promotional materials.

### economic and industrial understanding
- identification of new markets
- assessment of market potential
- the economic requirements of a profitable business.

## Useful Resource Tasks

**To enable students to analyse products to inform their designing and making:**
- SRT 5 *Attribute analysis*
- SRT 6 *Evaluating using ranking, preference and difference tests*
- SRT 8 *User trip and performance specification*
- SRT 9 *Evaluation by attribute profile.*

**To enable students to develop high-quality making skills:**
- SRT 6 *Evaluating using ranking, preference and difference tests.*

**To enable students to consider small batch production issues:**
- FPRT 1 *Batch production and systems thinking.*

**To enable students to develop promotion for a product range:**
- CRT 1 *Presenting information about food products.*

## Useful Case Studies

**To develop an understanding of bread products:**
- Breadmaking in Peru
- Bread production.

## Design brief

To design and make a range of specialized bread products to be made and sold by a small family business bakery and develop appropriate promotion.

## Preliminary specification

**What the product should do:**
- be based on bread
- offer an original new taste and texture and may be either sweet or savoury.

**What the product should look like:**
- have a distinctive appearance throughout the range.

**Other features:**
- be capable of being stored for one to two days without undue deterioration
- be promoted as meeting healthy eating requirements.

## Possible associated activities

- visit a bakery or watch a video to see production processes
- interview the baker at a small bakery to identify the problems of market competition
- compare the products in the baker's shop to those in the supermarket
- investigate and test the range of ingredients available for making bread
- carry out tests on storage.

## Design sketches

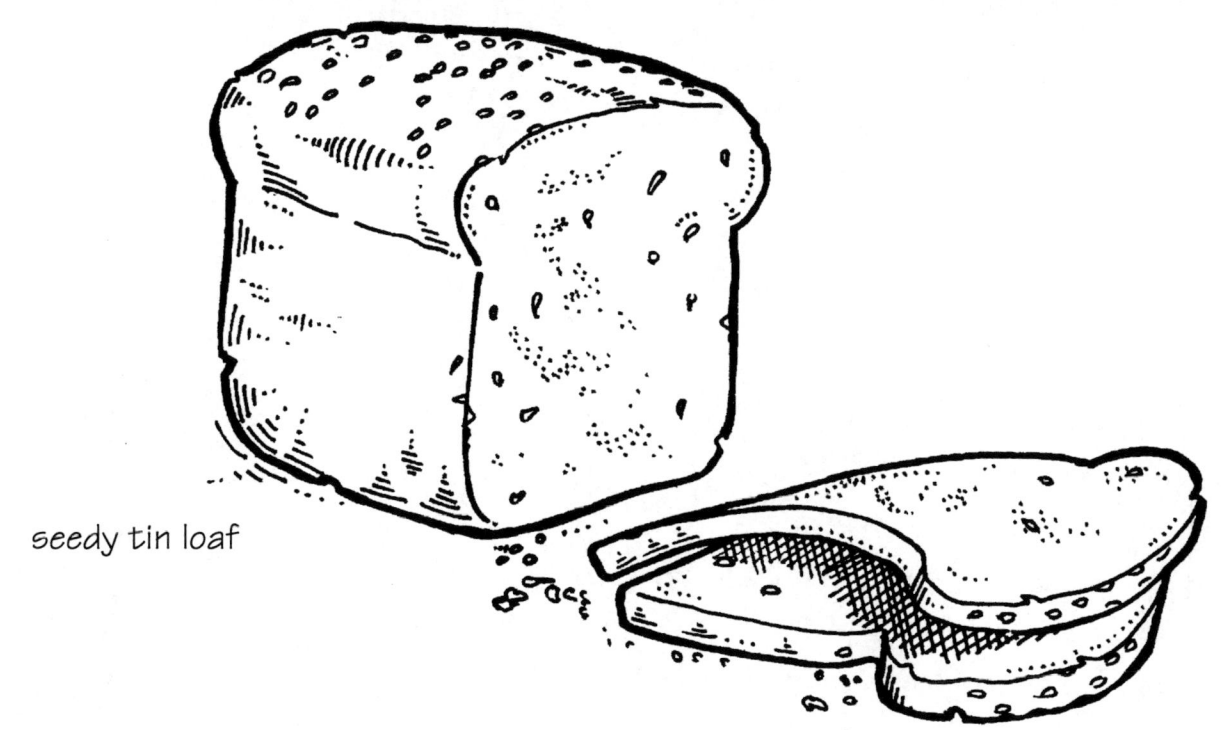

seedy tin loaf

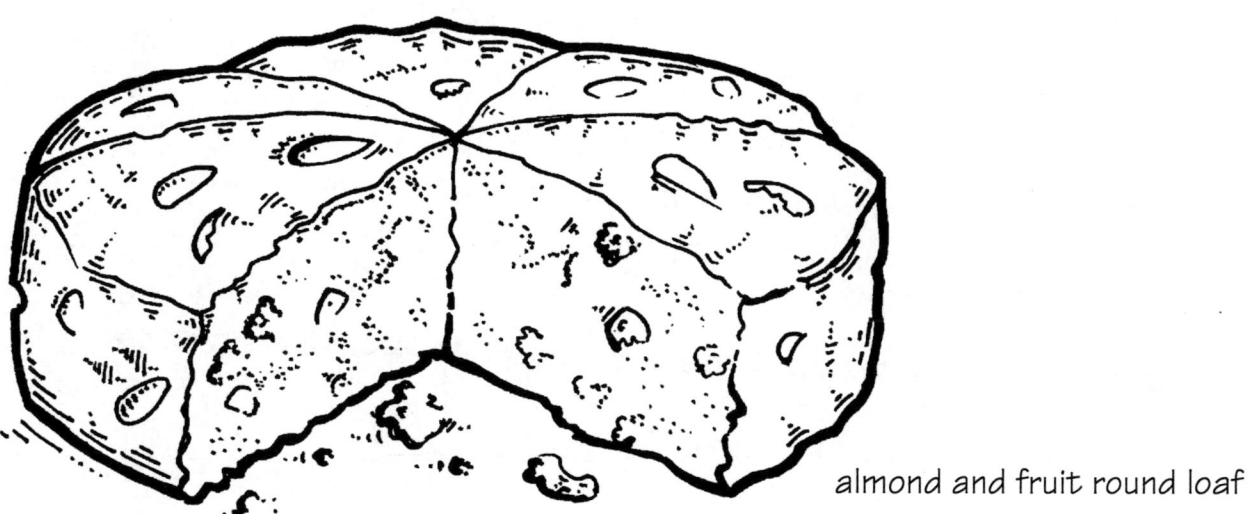

almond and fruit round loaf

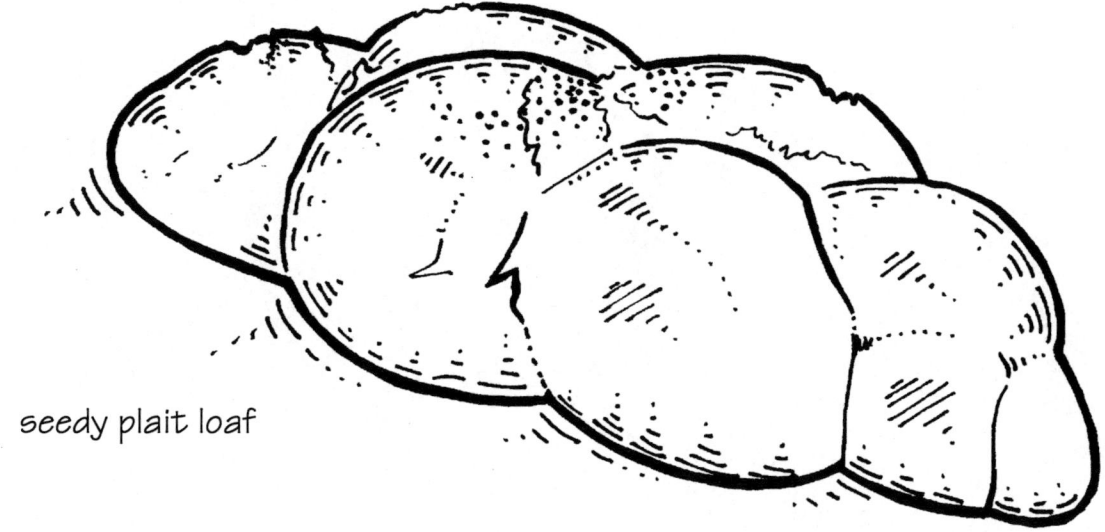

seedy plait loaf

# Kitchen Garden Plait

**Ingredients:**

500 g granary flour
2 tablespoons of olive oil
6 g easy blend dried yeast
150 ml yeast
1 teaspoon of chopped fresh herbs
25 g of grated Leicester cheese

**Method:**

1 Sieve warmed flour, add yeast, herbs and olive oil. Add warmed milk and beat until the bowl becomes clean.

2 Turn on to lightly floured table and knead until smooth and springy to the touch.

3 Allow to prove in a warm place until the dough is doubled in size.

4 Turn on to table and re-knead.

5 Divide dough into 3 pieces. Roll each piece and plait.

6 Top with grated cheese. Allow to prove in a warm place until double in size.

7 Bake at oven mark 7 or 220°C for 15 to 20 mins.

# Better than a sandwich

## A Capability Task for food technology
### Line of interest – food products from the bakery

## The task

To design and make a range of bread-based snack lunch alternatives to sandwiches.

## Task setting

A small family business bakery already sells home-made breads, cakes and biscuits, but has identified a potential, multicultural, local market for ready prepared snack lunch products.

## The aims of the task

- to enable students to analyse products to inform their designing and making
- to enable students to explore markets
- to develop an understanding of bread products
- to enable students to develop high-quality making skills and consider small batch production issues
- to enable students to develop promotion for a product range.

## Values

### technical
Students should consider the need for hazard analysis and quality control during food processing and production.

### economic
Students should consider the contribution specialized products make to the overall profitability of a small business.

### aesthetic
Students should consider the visual aspects of food products that might be derived from cultural influences.

### moral
Students should consider the impact of snack meals on the way we live.

### social
Students should consider the role of a small bakery in the life of a local community.

### environmental
Students should consider world issues of ingredient cultivation and development, together with the effects of manufacturing processes on the environment today.

## Nature of the product

### exploration
- a report on existing products to suit a variety of cultures
- a report on a visit to a bakery
- a report on the testing and analysis of consumer preferences for this food range
- consideration of the effects of storage and reheating on possible food products
- a preliminary specification for a new product

### production and promotion
- a report on suitable production systems
- a report on the suitability of identified food products
- a detailed specification for the final product, including ingredients, equipment and a production schedule
- sample products
- promotional material

### possible products
- filled naan breads
- pasties/samosas with various fillings
- special diet pastry or bread products.

## Technical knowledge and understanding

- knowledge of sensory analysis
- knowledge of a variety of multicultural methods used to produce breads and pastries
- knowledge of dietary requirements of a snack meal product
- knowledge of dietary analysis of ingredients and their value to the consumer
- knowledge of the suitability of batch production systems.

© The Nuffield Foundation, 1996

## Specialist tools, materials and equipment

- a wide range of flours
- food processors with dough-kneading accessories
- microwave ovens.

## Cross-curricular links

### maths

- accurate measurement, calculating nutritional values, ratios for portion sizes.

### science

- relevant concepts – raising agents as chemical reactions that generate gases.

### art

- analysis of form to generate the shapes of bread products.

### IT

- use of spreadsheets for costing and nutritional analysis
- use of DTP for reports and promotional materials.

### economic and industrial understanding

- identification of new markets
- assessment of market potential
- the economic requirements of a profitable business.

## Useful Resource Tasks

**To enable students to explore markets:**
- SRT 2 *Questionnaires*
- SRT 4 *Brainstorming*.

**To enable students to analyse products to inform their designing and making:**
- SRT 6 *Evaluating using ranking, preference and difference tests*
- SRT 8 *User trip and performance specification*
- SRT 9 *Evaluation by attribute profile*.

**To enable students to develop high-quality making skills:**
- SRT 6 *Evaluating using ranking, preference and difference tests*.

**To enable students to consider small batch production issues:**
- FPRT 1 *Batch production and systems thinking*.

**To enable students to develop promotion for a product range:**
- CRT 1 *Presenting information about food products*.

## Useful Case Studies

**To develop an understanding of bread products:**
- Breadmaking in Peru
- Bread production.

## Design brief

To design and make a savoury snack lunch product that might be made and sold by a small local bakery and develop appropriate promotion for it. It may be eaten cold or reheated and should satisfy the lunchtime needs of a multicultural working community.

## Preliminary specification

**What the product should do:**
- provide an individual lunch portion that can be eaten without cutlery.

**What the product should look like:**
- have a distinctive appearance across the range.

**Other features:**
- may be eaten hot or cold
- be part of a range that appeals to different cultural groups
- be promoted as meeting healthy eating requirements.

## Possible associated activities

- visit a bakery or watch a video to see production processes
- interview the baker at a small bakery to identify the problems of market competition
- compare the products in bakers' shops to those in supermarkets
- analyse the dietary value of existing products.

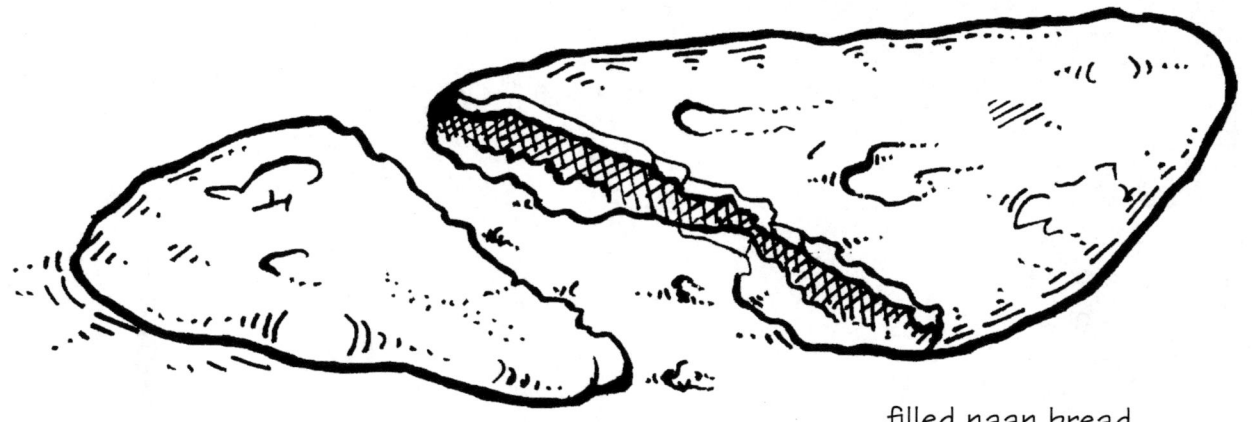

filled naan bread

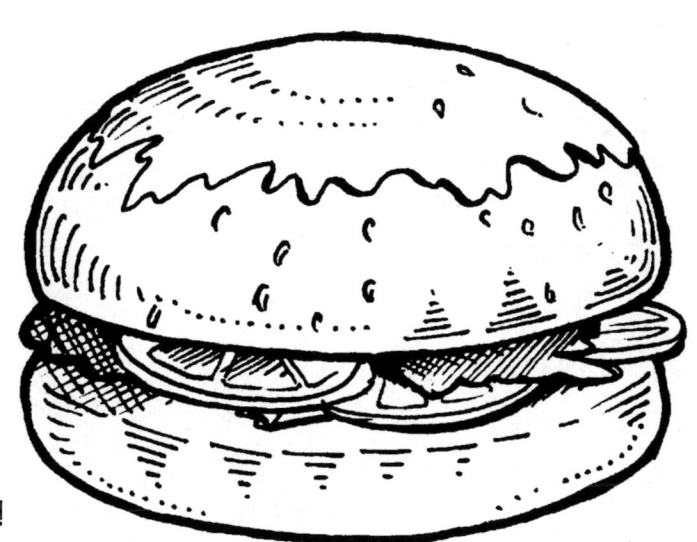

the traditional burger!

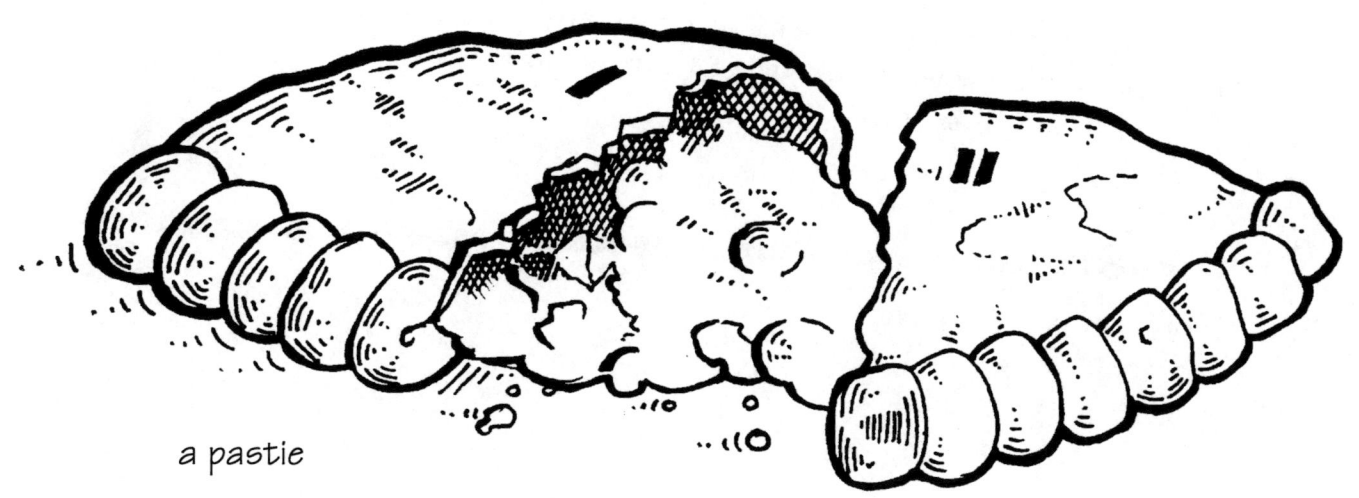

a pastie

# Tandoori Chicken Pastie

**Ingredients:**
500 g strong white flour
25 g margarine
6 g easy blend dried yeast
150 ml water

**Filling:**
2 chicken breasts

**Marinade:**
1 tablespoon Dijon mustard
100 ml oil
100 ml natural yoghurt
10 g fresh chopped ginger
1/2 teaspoon of cumin, coriander seeds and ground turmeric combined
juice of 1/2 small lemon

**Method:**

1 Prepare marinade for chicken by combining ingredients carefully.

2 Remove skin from chicken, rub and cover with marinade. Leave to stand for at least 6 hours. Grill for about 15 mins on each side. Cool.

3 Sieve warmed flour, add yeast and rubbed in margarine. Add warmed milk and beat until the bowl becomes clean.

4 Turn on to lightly floured table and knead until smooth and springy to the touch.

5 Allow to prove in a warm place until the dough is doubled in size.

6 Turn on to table and re-knead. Shape into circles for pasties, fill, seal, sprinkle with sesame seeds. Allow to prove in a warm place for 10 mins, until double in size.

7 Bake in oven mark 7 or 220°C for 10 to 15 mins.

# Luxury cakes （11）

## The task

To design and make a range of individual (one or two portions), boxed, decorated, luxury cakes with maximum keeping qualities.

## Task setting

A school mini-enterprise scheme has the aim of generating funds for a chosen charity or need. The students' task is to design and make a range of luxury, decorated cakes, each with their own identity, to meet the needs of numerous kinds of celebration around the world. The cakes must be suitable for mass production. Each cake is to be suitably packaged to promote the product and extend its shelf-life.

## The aims of the task

- to enable students to explore different celebrations and to include regional, cultural and religious themes
- to enable students to investigate different types and ratios of cake ingredients and their potential keeping qualities
- to enable students to consider the most suitable and successful materials for decorative purposes

- to enable students to consider food safety and hygiene when designing products that have to be transported and have a long shelf-life
- to enable students to develop appropriate packaging design and promotional material.

## Values

### technical
Students should consider the degree of precision required for quality luxury confectionery.

### economic
Students should consider the market for specialized luxury items.

### aesthetic
Students should consider the extent to which the appearance of a celebratory luxury product and its packaging contribute to its success.

### moral
Students should consider the worth of producing luxury food products that only a few people can afford.

### social
Students should consider the range of celebrations that are experienced and enjoyed in a multicultural society.

### environmental
Students should consider the need to minimize packaging without compromising protection or visual appeal.

## Nature of the product

### exploration
- a report on different sorts of party/celebration, associated confectionery and the possibilities for product development
- a report on a visit to a confectioners
- a report on the testing and analysis of the possible ingredients and methods of processing
- a preliminary specification for a new product

### production and promotion
- a report on suitable production systems
- a report on the product development, evaluated against the product specification
- a detailed specification for the final product that includes ingredients, equipment and a production schedule
- packaging and promotional material

### possible products
- small cakes made using a variety of methods – creamed, rubbed in, whisked, melted
- flavour enhanced by a variety of methods – spices, fruit, honey
- shaped by a variety of methods – moulding, cutting, layering, rolling
- decorated by a variety of methods – spun sugar, butter icing, sugar icing, marzipan, chocolate.

## Technical knowledge and understanding

- knowledge and understanding of the different cake making methods
- knowledge and understanding of the behaviour of different decorative materials

- knowledge of the suitability of batch production systems
- knowledge of food safety and hygiene regulations for cakes and packaging.

© The Nuffield Foundation, 1996

## Specialist tools, materials and equipment

- food mixers and processors
- tins (home-made from baked bean tins).

## Cross-curricular links

### maths
- nets for protective packaging.

### science
- relevant concepts – raising agents as chemical reactions that generate gases; the formation of foams.

### art
- the different styles of decoration used by different cultures.

### IT
- use of DTP to produce reports and promotion materials.

### economic and industrial understanding
- identification of new markets
- assessment of market potential
- the economic requirements of a profitable business.

## Useful Resource Tasks

**To enable students to explore different celebrations, including regional, cultural and religious themes:**
- SRT 1 *Identifying needs and likes*
- SRT 2 *Questionnaires*
- SRT 7 *Winners and losers and appropriateness*
- SRT 8 *User trip and performance specification.*

**To enable students to consider the most suitable and successful materials for decorative purposes:**
- DFPRT 5 *Designing for finish.*

**To enable students to consider food safety and hygiene when designing products that have to be transported and to have a long shelf-life:**
- FSRT 1 *Breaking the chain.*

**To enable students to develop appropriate packaging design and promotional materials:**
- CRT 1 *Presenting information about food products.*

## Useful Case Studies

- Embedded energy.

**To enable students to consider food safety and hygiene when designing products that have to be transported and to have a long shelf-life:**
- Wrap it up.

## Design brief

To design and make a range of individual (one or two portions), boxed, decorated, luxury cakes with maximum keeping qualities to meet identified celebration needs.

## Preliminary specification

**What the product should do:**
- be a luxury, cake-based confectionery item suitable for parties and celebrations.

**What the product should look like:**
- be extremely attractive and in keeping with the nature of the party or celebration.

**Other features:**
- individual product of one or two small portions
- packaged to extend its shelf-life (to a minimum of three weeks)
- the packaging should promote the product.

## Possible associated activities

- visit a confectioners to see production processes
- interview the confectioner to identify the problems of packaging and shelf-life
- investigate and test the range of methods and ingredients available for making cake-based products
- carry out investigations into packaging to extend shelf-life.

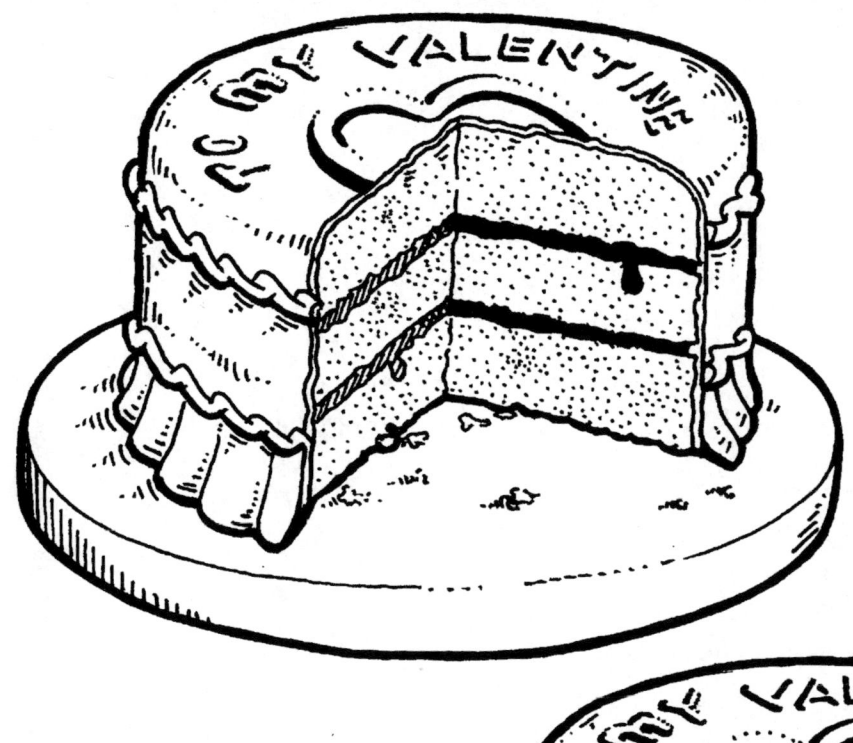

a Valentine's Day cake inside
and out, and in its box

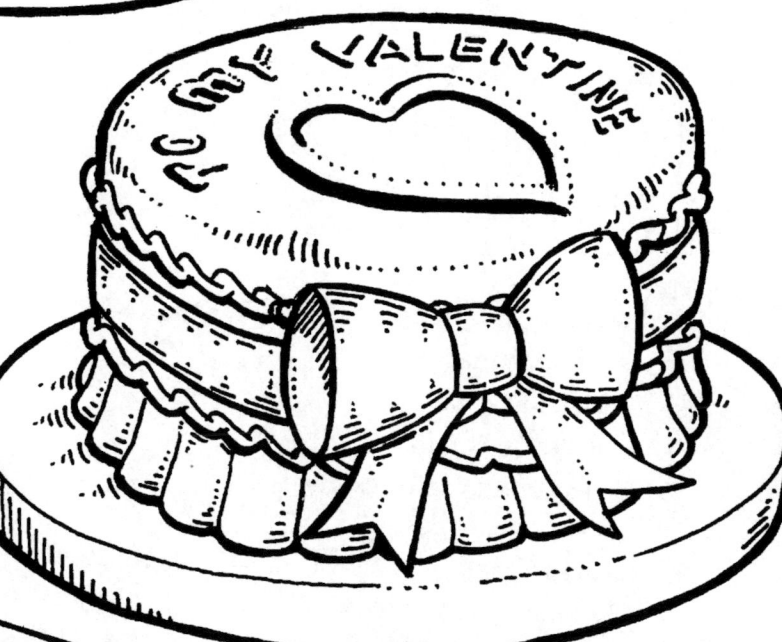

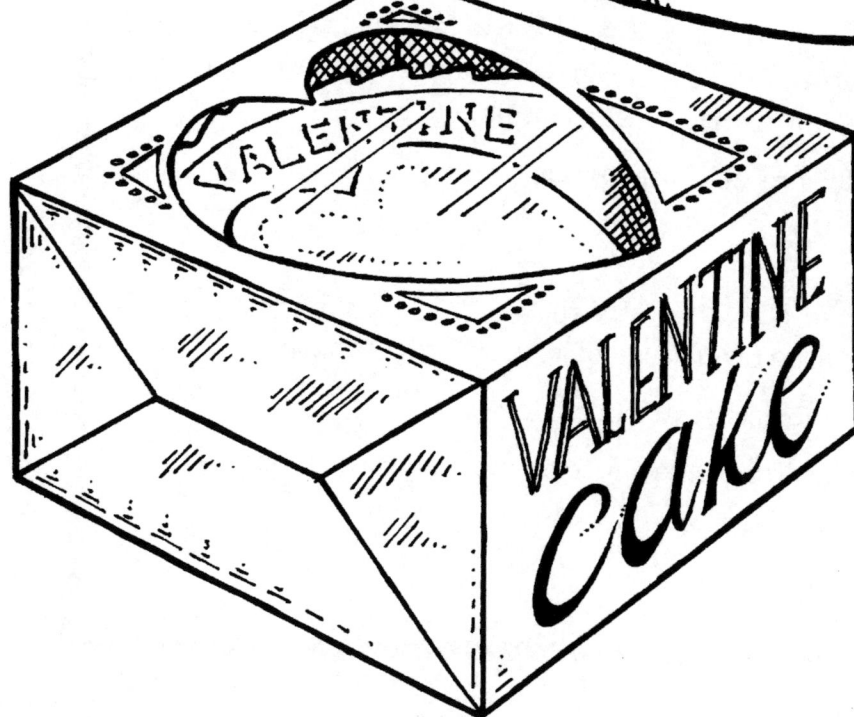

# St Valentine's Day Cake

**Ingredients:**

350 g soft margarine
75 g self-raising flour
50 g oats

250 g caster sugar
25 g drinking chocolate
3 large eggs

**Method:**

1 Oven mark 4 or 180°C. Grease and line with greaseproof paper 3 x 12-13 cm sandwich tins.

2 Cream margarine and sugar until soft and creamy.

3 Beat in eggs half at a time.

4 Fold carefully combined flour, oats and drinking chocolate.

5 Bake for 15 to 20 mins until firm to the touch.

6 Turn out and cool.

**Filling:**

Strawberry jam

**Vanilla butter icing:**

75 g butter/margarine
225 g icing sugar
2 tablespoons milk
1/4 teaspoon vanilla essence

**Method:**

Place ingredients in bowl and beat well.

**Fondant icing:**

350 g icing sugar
1 medium egg white
1 tablespoon liquid glucose
2 drops pink colouring (for heart)

**Method:**

1 Blend all ingredients together.
2 Knead well to form a pliable ball on a clean work surface. Dredge lightly with cornflour.

Either melted chocolate or royal icing for piping writing
Red ribbon and cake board

**Decorating the cake:**

1 Sandwich 3 cakes together with layers of jam and butter icing.

2 Cover thinly with butter icing and fondant icing.

3 Cut out a heart for top in pink fondant icing and pipe message on cake.

4 Tie red ribbon around cake.

5 Package.

# Confectionery by post (12)

## The task

To design and make a range of personalized luxury confectionery items suitable for parties and celebrations.

## Task setting

A mail order design company wants to produce a catalogue of designs of personalized luxury confectionery items. The products in the catalogue must be suitable for mass production and be packaged in a way that protects the products during transportation. The design company will publish the promotional material and offer a design service for special events.

## The aims of the task

- to enable students to explore different sorts of party and celebration and include regional, cultural and religious themes
- to enable students to explore the needs and opportunities for sugar-based products in relation to designing a luxury item
- to enable students to develop an understanding of relevant food chemistry

- to enable students to consider food safety and hygiene when designing products that have to be transported and have a long shelf-life
- to enable students to develop appropriate packaging design and promotional material.

## Values

### technical
Students should consider the degree of precision required for quality confectionery.

### economic
Students should consider the market for specialized luxury items.

### aesthetic
Students should consider the cultural and other influences that might affect the appearance of personalized luxury confectionery items.

### moral
Students should consider the worth of producing luxury food products that only a few people can afford.

### social
Students should consider the role of celebration and parties in people's lives.

### environmental
Students should consider the materials used in the packaging of the product.

## Nature of the product

### exploration
- a report on different sorts of party/celebration, associated confectionery and possibilities for product development
- a report on a visit to a confectioners
- a report on the testing and analysis of the possible ingredients and methods of processing
- a preliminary specification for a new product

### possible products
- shaped and decorated sweets – fudge, toffees, chocolates, fondant, chocolate-covered preserved or dried fruits
- shaped and decorated biscuits
- shaped and decorated marzipan
- shaped and decorated ice-creams.

### production and promotion
- a report on suitable production systems
- a report on the product development and an evaluation of it with regard to the product specification
- a detailed specification for the final product, including ingredients, equipment and a production schedule
- packaging and promotional material

## Technical knowledge and understanding

- knowledge and understanding of the recipes for fudge, toffee, biscuits, marzipan, fondant, ice-cream
- knowledge and understanding of the behaviour of chocolate and sugar icing

- knowledge of the suitability of batch production systems
- knowledge of vacuum forming for mould production.

## Specialist tools, materials and equipment

- ice-cream maker
- access to modelling clay and vacuum former
- access to CNC milling machine for producing surface stamps.

## Cross-curricular links

### maths

- measuring to minimize waste while developing a production system.

### science

- relevant concepts – structure and properties of foams and emulsions.

### art

- the different styles of decoration used by different cultures.

### IT

- use of DTP to produce reports and promotion materials
- use of image manipulating software and CNC software to develop surface stamps.

### economical and industrial understanding

- identification of new markets
- assessment of market potential
- the economic requirements of a profitable business.

## Useful Resource Tasks

To enable students to explore different sorts of party and celebration, to include regional, cultural and religious themes:
- SRT 1 *Identifying needs and likes*
- SRT 2 *Questionnaires*
- SRT 7 *Winners and losers and appropriateness*
- SRT 8 *User trip and performance specification.*

To enable students to develop an understanding of relevant food chemistry:
- FCRT 3 *Looking at foams*
- FCRT 4 *Looking at emulsions.*

To enable students to consider food safety and hygiene when designing products that have to be transported and to have a long shelf-life:
- FSRT 1 *Breaking the chain.*

To enable students to develop appropriate packaging design and promotional material:
- CRT 1 *Presenting information about food products.*

In addition, students may find DFPRT 5, *Designing for finish*, useful.

## Useful Case Studies

Public transport in London; background to the transport needed for mail order and local deliveries.

To enable students to explore the needs and opportunities for sugar-based products in relation to designing a luxury item:
- Brand names for sweeties
- Cool control.

## Design brief

To design and make a range of personalized luxury confectionery items suitable for parties and celebrations with packaging that enables them to be supplied via a local delivery or mail order service.

## Preliminary specification

**What the product should do:**
- provide a luxury confectionery item suitable for parties and celebrations.

**What the product should look like:**
- be extremely attractive and in keeping with the nature of the party or celebration.

**Other features:**
- personalized
- packaged for local delivery or mail order
- supported by a mail order catalogue.

## Possible associated activities

- visit a confectioners to see production processes
- interview the confectioner to identify the problems of local delivery and mail order
- investigate and test the range of ingredients available for making suitable products
- mould-making for vacuum forming
- carry out tests on packaging for protection.

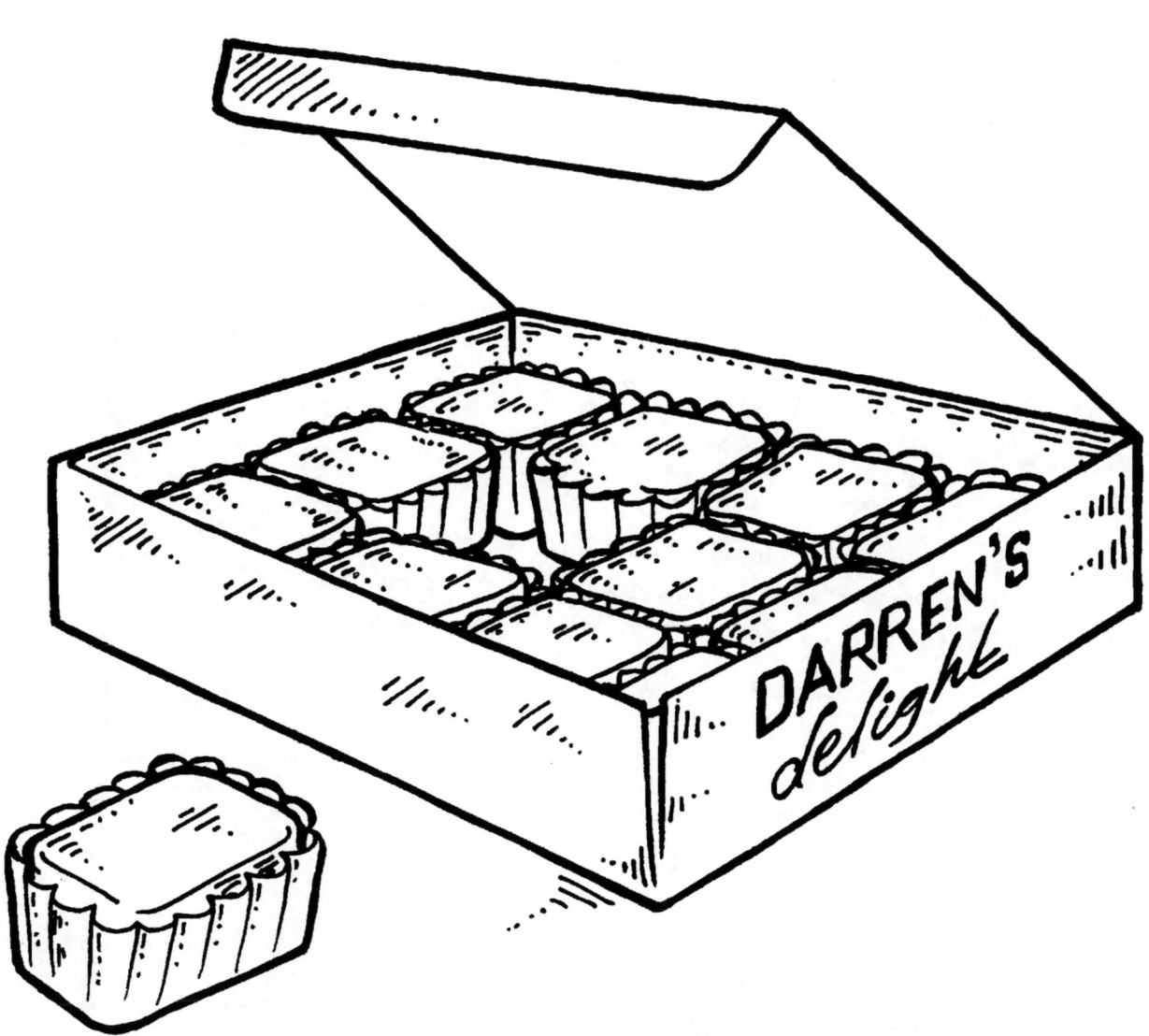

fudge by special delivery!

# Chocolate Fudge

**Ingredients:**

500 g sugar
150 ml milk
150 g butter/margarine
100 g plain chocolate
50 g clear honey

**Method:**

1 Place all the ingredients in heavy based saucepan

2 Stir over a low heat until dissolved.

3 Bring to the boil gently for about 10 mins to reach 118°C on a sugar thermometer. Test by dropping a little of the mixture into a cup of cold water. It will form a soft ball when rolled between the fingers.

4 Remove from heat immediately and cool base of pan on/in a cold surface/water.

5 Beat with a wooden spoon until the fudge becomes smooth in texture and thickens (grains).

6 Pour into a lightly oiled tin (20.5 x 15 cm). Mark into squares and cut when cold.